MENOPAUSE UNZIPPED

How to emerge as a goddess

By Freddy Carrick

First published April 2020

FOREWORD

The authentic empathy which Freddy has embedded into every chapter and story makes this book totally accessible to women of all ages.

I cannot wait to read this book, if only to gain a more complete understanding of what will happen to me when my perimenopause begins.

More importantly, I'll be having more discussions around oestrogen depletion with my colleagues and patients.

Aurora Almadori, MBBS, MSc, PhD

Table of Contents

COMING, READY OR NOT!

The menopause train is coming to a station near you, it's coming whether you're ready or not, if you were born female and are beyond puberty then it's already on the way.

For some of us it's an express train charging through all symptom-stations, never allowing the lack of air conditioning or effective sleep to slow it down; for others it's a cross country train that ponderously makes its way through every symptom-station including joint pain, hair loss and brain fog, before finally settling against the buffers of worn out old age. For many, this train will take a decade before it runs out of steam, but others will find they get on at one station, travel a brief distance before getting off to wander into a magnificent sunset with a beloved partner; the difference can be as simple as knowing what you don't know that you don't know, in other words, prepare for the best outcome by educating yourself.

Doesn't matter which ticket you have, you'll be climbing aboard a similar train at some point in your life, however much you want to avoid it. I've written this book for you, my sister, because I want to help in preparing you for the journey through menopause and into the most beautiful, fulfilling period of your life.

This is the book your mother, aunt, mentor, best friend or someone, should have given to you around your 42nd birthday. Why your 42nd? you'll find out soon. If you enjoy it and find it helpful, then make sure you buy it for every other female friend or relative you know who is under the age of 60.

In the UK, the average age of a female at menopause is 51; the average age of female suicide in the UK is 50-54. *Is this the ultimate hidden cost of a lack of menopause education, information, advice and support?*

If that fact worries you then you need to read and pay attention to the steps you can take to ensure you enjoy an easier and more supported menopause.

At time of writing this I'd like to offer grateful thanks to the female broadcasters and media stars who are gliding gracefully into their early fifties and talking, writing and making documentaries about the menopause. I'd like to pay tribute to every one of them who chooses to speak publicly about this change in their lives so that other women are encouraged to bring menopause into everyday conversation. Since the 1980's these women have been smashing glass ceilings and never allowing their femininity to stand in the way of competing with male colleagues.

That group of women aren't ready to 'bow out' of their prestigious positions just because their hormones have become unglued, and you shouldn't either. There are so many ways that women can remain strong and empowered throughout their lives, so let's not allow something like hormone changes to trip us up. I've written this book because I come into contact with dozens of women who are over 40 and are struggling in their lives because of unrecognised menopause symptoms.

While I'm not a health care professional, I am a woman of age and grace, and I know how it feels to lose the crutches of self-worth and confidence. I'm in my mid-sixties and I can clearly see that the midlife of the average woman could be improved immensely if only she understood why her body is behaving the way it is and what she can do to feel physically better, happier and more confident.

My intention is to help you understand what you can do to feel better and live a happier, less stressful and more energetic life during the years around your menopause. How many years will that be, I don't know and neither do you. I'd like to help you understand what symptoms you may be having and what you can do to relieve those symptoms. The thing is that all women are different and just because a female you know had certain symptoms it doesn't mean that you'll have them too, so this is a guide, a helpful book. It isn't a textbook or a set of rules that you should follow.

I must have written this book three times, and some chapters around 7 times. The more I wrote the more I researched, the more I learnt, the more I had to write.

Because I wanted this book to be easy to read and understand, a warm and friendly hug from one post-menopausal woman to all her sisters. I picked up too many books written by doctors and nurses which rarely offered true insight or helpful remedies but were full of facts.

I wrote and researched and re-wrote because I want and hope that you'll get such a great understanding you'll be able and willing to pass on all the information to your friends and family. The time to stop the silent suffering of women entering the perimenopause and menopause is long past. I believe it's shameful that so few medical professionals, from nurses to consultants, have any real understanding of women's health during this lengthy period which happens for every single female.

Tell your daughters ladies and let us spread the information far and wide so that the generations following will flow into and out of their menopause with ease and wonderful health. More importantly, the number of women in menopause who initiate divorce is growing; there is a great deal within this book to help those women at the end of their tether.

As a final note, there is ongoing research into the effect that overworked adrenal glands have on your body during life around the years of menopause. Look out for more information on the findings of this research on my website and blog.

INTRODUCTION

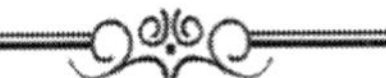

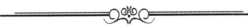

Menopause Unzipped will dispel the slew of mythology surrounding menopause. I will walk you through all the symptoms, using my personal stories and anecdotal stories from other women and medical professionals. I discuss everything from depression to vaginal problems, relationships (friends and partners) including how to keep everyone on side, and especially the emotional tsunami which can overwhelm in an instant. I will help you to overcome any fears you hold surrounding menopause and how your life will be afterwards.

My research into remedies is current and based on International Guidance on the Treatment of Menopausal Symptoms. (In UK our healthcare is free, and menopause is included, but I'm not sure about countries where all healthcare is insurance based, therefore some people may have menopause treatments included and others may not.)

After reading this book I hope you'll be more open about the menopause and stop treating it like a nightmare that never ends, or the end of femininity. Learn how to manage symptoms and other aspects, so you can flow onwards from it as a beautiful creature instead of feeling like washed out rags. I hope to dispel the idea that taking a prescription for hormone therapy isn't failing or giving in, and to discuss why it isn't. I go through the difference between prescription and over the counter remedies, educating you on safety and choosing best products.

I also want to enable and empower so that you can have an equal discussion with a doctor when you choose to discuss your symptoms, and to understand all options available to resolve them. Finally, I discuss how the symptoms develop and change as you age from early forties to late sixties and beyond.

Why

are mothers not educating their daughters about menopause?

Most mothers leave the education of daughters to a later date or never, a little like motherhood or making a souffle, skills to learn only when it becomes necessary. If I had a daughter, I would be educating her from her early 40s on what to expect and how to best manage her symptoms, but I've honestly never been told by a woman that her mother did this.

It's very common these days for women to begin their family later in life, so that by the time perimenopause arrives their children are barely teenagers. Imagine having to deal with pubescent teenagers and a husband working long hours, throw in some elderly parents who need care (all living longer than ever), and it isn't a surprise that many women just don't have the time to research their own healthcare, let alone make informed decisions.

Why

do women think that taking hormone therapy through menopause has terrifying side effects?

do women think that hormone therapy only masks the menopause and once you stop taking it the symptoms all begin again?

do women think they have to put up with menopause symptoms because 'it's just their age'?

are only 50% of British women going to see a GP or nurse about their menopause symptoms, even though their symptoms are having a significant and negative affect on their functioning, performance, confidence, relationships and sex life?

do so many women choose to ignore their symptoms until they're on the brink of murder, divorce, losing their job or, heaven help them, thinking about ending their life?

do women choose to focus on the alleged detrimental effects of supplementing their hormones via medication, rather than focus on how that supplementation can benefit their life and health?

do so many women not understand the perimenopause, its symptoms and the remedies available, when this happens to every single female on this planet; therefore, there are forests of magazine and newspaper articles? There are books and blogs and Facebook groups, and internet pages by the thousand.

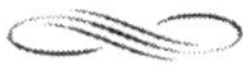

Why

do you only chat about 'menopause brain' in a self-derogatory way, making a joke of it? Are you afraid that talking openly about your symptoms makes you 'not up to the job'? It's true that your memory isn't what it used to be and if you're in a job requiring terrific organisational skills, then you may feel that you're failing on some days.

do you feel that telling someone how sad you feel about your loss of fertility will make you look pathetic?

are women ashamed of being in hormonal transition? Is it because very few people have any understanding of it, and this includes our family, partners, even most health care professionals, it's sad to say?

I'm going to answer all of these questions in later chapters.

> **Perhaps**
>
> it's because to admit to being in the menopause acknowledges that a woman is around 50 years old, and the discussion could place her at a disadvantage in the workplace and perhaps, past it. I believe there is a trend within modern workplaces to make attempts to support women who are going through menopause, those HR departments need to be applauded.

After you read this book, when it's your turn to collect that train ticket to perimenopause city, you won't be surprised. Around 20% of women living in the western world will barely notice any changes in their body apart from a bit of weight gain, good for them I say. Don't just hope that you'll be one of them, BE PREPARED in case you're not.

My intention is to help you understand what you can do to feel better and live a happier, less stressful **and more energetic life** during the years around your menopause. How many years will that be, I don't know and neither do you. I'd like to help you understand what symptoms you may be having and what you can do to relieve those symptoms. The thing is that all women are different and just because a female you know had certain symptoms it doesn't mean that you'll have them too, so this is a guide, a helpful book. It isn't a textbook or a set of rules that you should follow.

So, let's dive in

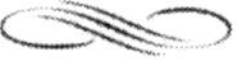

Part One of this book will look at all the symptoms of peri and post menopause, what they are, the effect they might have on your life and how they develop through the different stages of menopause. You will never again need to ask "why am I feeling like this" when you find yourself sitting in the car outside of the supermarket because you can't face going in.

If you feel confusion, outrage, disbelief, ignorant or insulted should any of your family suggest you might be entering menopause, you're not alone. There is a sense of shame among women around the idea of being 'that age' and it truly is so sad. Women are totally disadvantaged by hormones from puberty till they die, and it's just not fair.

I'm going to educate you that perimenopause symptoms are likely to be felt from early 40s, so that you won't spend two or three years wondering if you're suffering early onset dementia, or having a nervous breakdown, or thinking that you've become moody and selfish when it comes to looking after yourself.

During research for this book I've spoken to many friends in their forties; they told me about feeling fat, forgetful, emotional, disorganised, tired, and many other complaints. Every time I asked them their age and suggested they might be in perimenopause, they looked at me slightly offended, laughed and said 'crikey, I'm not that old'. This is what I want you to understand; in the 21st century, early 40s is not old, but it is the approximate age when your body begins its final hormonal transition.

In 2012 Oprah Winfrey published some conversations on her YouTube channel around menopause. In the UK, an open discussion via TV, radio, and many publications has begun this last year, with media personalities such as Kay Burley, Mariella Frostrup, Andrea McLean and Carol Vorderman all fully disclosing how they manage their own menopause. Hopefully the conversation won't stop, and our young female relatives will get the message that menopause isn't to be feared and no woman is old just because her fertility ends.

However; in 2019, most women I speak to who are over 40 still don't understand what is going to happen to their bodies because of hormones, and what can be done about it. My education around menopause was extremely casual, and all I understood was it would 'happen' when I was in my fifties. I knew that my periods would stop, and I would probably have to deal with embarrassing hot flushes.

I had absolutely no idea of this stretch of time called the perimenopause, or that it would indicate the slowing down of oestrogen production during which the diminished hormone could cause havoc through all of my systems, creating mental and physical lethargy, memory lapse, hot flushes and a long list of other symptoms.

Are women ashamed of being in hormonal transition?

Part Two will look at all the remedies that I have discovered, and how they can help with symptoms. I'm going to discuss remedies available in health food stores, pharmacies and within the complimentary health professions. I intend to provide as much information as I can so that you can make the best decision about what's right for you. Everyone's menopause is different, so don't listen to other people who tell you that you should be doing this or should be doing that. Let them should all over themselves and have their own experiences and results. Your menopause is unique, live it your way.

Of the hundreds of Facebook posts and comments I've read and the dozens of women I interviewed, not a single one of them has said "I buy sage leaves, black cohosh, wild yam, soy supplements, red clover, CBD oil, flax seeds, or whatever, every month and *I got my life back"*. Nor have any of them told me that they paid for private aromatherapy, reflexology, EFT, herbology advice, nutritional advice, and their days are relatively symptom free.

Unlike the posts from women who have found a doctor who understands menopause or who have paid privately for a specialist. Perhaps it took them two or three tries, but they found the right combination of oestrogen, progesterone, and testosterone supplements in the right format (gel/pill/patch or suppository); those women do post **I'm on HRT and I got my life back.**

Which is why I am definitely pro pharmaceutical intervention, if only because this stage of your life is too darned important to ignore the most effective and powerful remedies available as soon as you need them. I also understand that there is a deal of cynicism and caution surrounding the intentions and integrity of some pharmaceutical companies.

I do understand that in some countries the cost of HRT is prohibitive which is why women have little choice but to go down the alternative route.

My reasons for going through all of the remedies is that you need to think about how you will manage whatever symptoms you face and be prepared to change your mind when or if they happen. Just as in childbirth, many women declare they don't want any pain relief until the baby enters the birth canal, many change their mind.

I'm unequivocally on the side of taking a pragmatic view of the menopause and of doing whatever is necessary to ensure your family and career don't suffer because of it. That's why I've written a lot about supporting your body through this change by blowing a bit of wind beneath your wings in the form of very gentle hormone replacement.

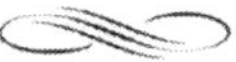

Goddess Academy is what we're here for, and in this part, I'll be sharing the reasons why, at 67, I'm a figure of inspiration among a Community of high achievers.

My chapters within the Goddess Academy cover major life events, leadership, resilience, (emotional) behaviours and more. We're going to explore my version of a goddess in the 21st Century; how she looks and behaves, what her values and beliefs might be and how she can thrive in this world. This is nothing to do with spirituality or having any 'mystical' skills particularly but is all about how she lives her life and manages her relationships.

Some women will be happy being able to get out of bed every day and function well, leaving the goddess part to someone else. Choices.

Let's change the unspoken acceptance that the last third of a woman's life is irrelevant or embarrassing just because her body is performing its own version of hormonal magic. It's unfortunate that this type of magic can be debilitating on many levels, potentially putting women at professional disadvantage.

AND, let's discuss the monumental celebration we should enjoy during this 'rite of passage'.

With knowledge comes power, so we should share information a lot more often in the workplace. We should expect our employers to look beyond the wrinkles and appreciate the woman who often works harder than most men, just because she feels a need to prove her worth. Employers need to provide more than an occasional lunchtime talk in the staff room and a desk fan to support their female employees. I would urge you to become a leader at work and educate your employers.

PART ONE

I'M NOT THAT OLD!

Is the glass ceiling that holds women back from true greatness really called menopause?

These scenarios have happened either to me or to a friend. These sneaky unexpected tweaks to our normal operational behaviour can derail the whole train, making us feel just a bit lost.

Your life is great, career's going well, children are happy and busy taking exams; partner is busy building the pension pot. Last year you helped your parents downsize because Dad can't manage the stairs so well and they needed a smaller garden. Everyone is ok and you manage to keep all the plates spinning with flair, being the person others can depend on gives you a feeling of satisfaction and fulfilment.

One day you realise that you forgot the name of your favourite actor while discussing his latest movie, and it's not the first time. Yesterday you put the sugar bowl in the fridge and after a ten-minute frantic search of your house for the car keys, they turned up in the cutlery drawer.

Sitting at your computer you go to create a new spreadsheet and can't remember how it works, or even your name! The stress of these memory lapses brings on a sweat around your hairline and top lip, which moves down your neck and you begin to feel hot between your breasts. Realising your colleagues have noticed your flush, you hesitate and stop speaking. Disappear to the ladies' room for a freshen up, but it happens again later that day.

Walking out to the car with no time to spare because you are never late for appointments, you feel a familiar rush of warmth between your legs and realise you weren't expecting your period today. Rushing back inside you barely reach the bathroom before your panties are soaked and it just doesn't seem to stop. You plug with a tampon, slap the heaviest sanni pad available into your fresh panties and head out of the door, fingers crossed that you'll arrive in time to change yourself again before your appointment. It isn't the first time this heavy bleed has happened unexpectedly, but your periods are all over the place these last few months and you don't know when to expect them.

Getting ready for a night out which you planned weeks ago and have been looking forward to catching up with your best girlfriends. As you dry your hair, you're getting upset because it just won't do what it normally does when you offer up the brush and hair dryer routine. You can see your scalp where the hair parts at the front, and it just doesn't bounce the way it used to. You begin to feel frustrated because your hair is a major factor in your 'look', and if it isn't right then nothing looks right. Beginning to feel hot and flustered, you can't remember if you put the gel on already. When you told a friend about it last week, she said that when this happened to her sister, the sister went straight to the hairdresser and had it all chopped short and spiky. That really frightened you because your shoulder length waves have always been glorious and you don't want to change. Surely this is just because you changed your conditioner and maybe you don't need to use so much. Next time you go to the hairdresser for your colour, you'll mention this lack of bounce and see what she suggests.

Wandering around the local boutique you find some fabulous trousers at the right price in the perfect fabric for summer and try them on. The zip is difficult to fasten and the button at the top won't meet, so you check the size. It's your size, and the brand is the same as you usually buy. Try a bigger size in case the labels were wrong, and the waist fastens well, but the fit around the hips is too loose. Decide to not bother with trousers and look at lingerie instead because you noticed that your breasts are a bit bigger than your bra cup at present. Ask the assistant to measure you and discover that you need a bigger cup, happy days. However, none of your old bras fit anymore and that's an expensive replacement. The downside is that when you sit down there's an unexpected roll of flesh between breast and waistline, it completely ruins the silhouette, and now your favourite dress looks out of shape.

WHY WHY WHY? When you've been slim and fit for most of your adult life, even losing the weight of maternity fairly quickly, have you almost overnight, changed shape? Or why, when you've had fabulous curves do you now feel someone filled in your middle, now more apple than hourglass?

This chapter will explain all of the symptoms of perimenopause and menopause so that you know *why* and are prepared for the unexpected. I've also set this out in a simple chart form which you can easily refer to. Waft it in front of your partner and children and suggest that they give you more support around the home.

The menopause has many symptoms, a bit like the head of Medusa, and as stated elsewhere, that's because oestrogen maintains balance in almost all of our bodily systems. The slowing down of oestrogen production and its release causes those systems to go out of balance, which creates all of the symptoms explained.

A lot of women miss the first signs of menopause because they just aren't expecting it. We're educated to believe that we will be in menopause in our early 50s, but no one I've spoken to has been educated to understand that perimenopause (marking the slowing down of oestrogen production) starts in our early 40s. The first sign that your body is changing might be that you begin to have night sweats, or your periods change and become heavier or less regular. Those night sweats turn into daytime hot flushes and mood swings, intercourse is different, and you don't enjoy it as much. When you or someone who loves you points out that you 'don't seem yourself' then maybe it's time to think about perimenopause.

You may decide to visit your doctor because, even though you've never had premenstrual tension symptoms before, they suddenly develop in your mid-40's. Or if you do have regular PMS it becomes much worse, just like the irritability and irrationality of a teenager. You may become angry, paranoid, have panic attacks, or develop migraine attacks for the first time in your forties, as I did. The majority of women do not expect any of these symptoms until they are past the age of 50 and are expecting only two or three symptoms to last between 2-5 years, and then it will be over. Those expected symptoms are likely to be the most discussed ones, hot flushes, night sweats, sleep disturbance and perhaps mood swings.

If you had been told at school that menopause symptoms could last up to 12 years and might mean you would lose your husband, home, and lead you to give up the career you love, then you might have paid more attention.

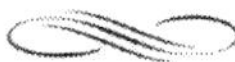

It's the transition from a relatively carefree life of eating well, enjoying wine with friends and partner, wearing what you like and perhaps sharing clothes with daughters. To the massive mental shift of the end of fertility and thinking it must mean that you're old. After all, when we were children our grandmothers (usually) looked 'old' and they must have been post-menopausal.

There's dreadful tiredness, or chronic fatigue, which feels as though your body simply closes down and your 'life force' has drained away, and you have to rest. One of the reasons for that is sleep deprivation caused by night sweats, and emotional turmoil caused by, well on some days it can be almost every single thing. If you've ever lived through emotional trauma, whatever the cause, you'll understand how physically exhausting it is.

Later, other symptoms arrive; there's a whole list of changes women don't talk about over a glass of wine, ranging from bed-wetting to dry vagina. You probably won't discuss those symptoms because you all think you're the only one with the problem. They can change your loving relationship from warm and intimate to frosty and don't come near me, overnight.

While researching this book, I had a thought that made me laugh out loud. Think about those horrid women in fairy tales; Cruella de Ville, The Queen in Snow White, Cinderella's stepmother; clearly menopausal women who were desperate to hold onto their youth and femininity. I'm sure you can think of several others who fit the description.

Many women manage their physical symptoms well but when they lose libido, drive and motivation, have no will to live, can no longer multitask and lose their ability to cope well with their complex lives, then they will hopefully look for the support of their doctor

Memory loss, brain fog, verbal mistakes and other cognitive effects of the perimenopause and menopause have caused many successful and senior businesswomen to give up work either because they simply couldn't cope any more or believed themselves to be 'losing their mind'.

Lots of women visit their doctor just to confirm what they're thinking; that they are, in fact, going through the menopause and not actually having a breakdown or developing some kind of disorder. Often, they simply want a conversation around the issues and to understand why they suddenly feel so different.

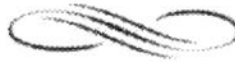

Unfortunately, and I can only speak about medical care in the UK, it is currently rare to find a health clinic or surgery where a member of the team specialises in or has an interest in menopause. During the writing of this book I spoke to many women at various stages of their menopause. Many of them were underwhelmed, or even distressed by the response from their doctor.

Sadly, some clinicians will listen to the list of symptoms and placate the patient with a 'well, it's that time of life', or 'you're sad because the children are leaving home', and 'I think you have a level of depression' (he looks at a Scale of Depression chart, tick, tick tick). This often results in women being given a prescription for anti-depressants to relieve anxiety or to aid sleep, and that just deepens her feeling of low self-worth or failure. Anti-depressant treatment can work well in the reduction of some symptoms, but it won't address the symptoms caused by lack of oestrogen. This is why I've written this book, to empower you to take charge of your own health and to be informed about your menopause.

Thankfully, the medical profession is waking up to the need to be better informed around menopause, and medical centres are improving the management of it. By the time you read this book, you should be able to speak to a doctor who has made it their speciality and will know all the information you need to hear.

The symptoms of menopause can be roughly divided into three groups; physical, emotional and sexual.

- **Physical symptoms** are hot flushes, night sweats, decreased bone density, hair changes, heartbeat changes, headaches, digestive changes, joint pain and stiffness, muscle tension or cramp, menstrual changes, skin changes, skin itching, weight gain, sleep disturbances, vaginal dryness, bladder incontinence, chronic tiredness
- **Emotional symptoms** are anxiety and stress, brain fog and poor concentration, depression, irritability, lack of focus, memory lapses, moodiness, overwhelm, panic attacks, thoughts of self-harm, suicidal thoughts,
- **Sexual symptoms** are loss of libido, lack of sexual pleasure, lack of interest in your loving partner

Let's have a look at all the above in more detail.

Please be aware that not everything that's changed in your physical and emotional being is because of peri menopause. Ovarian cancer is underdiagnosed and is regularly diagnosed late. If you have any of the above symptoms, then go and talk to your doctor or practice nurse and have a good and open conversation.

AGES & STAGES - TIME FOR A CHANGE

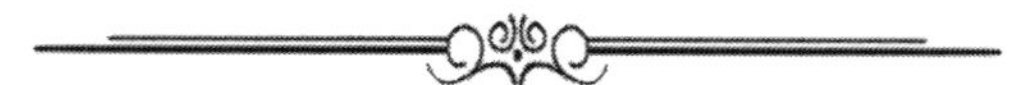

This too shall pass

You want and need to know which symptoms to expect from your menopause, and when to expect them. Given that all women are different, this is a simple guide.

Premenopause is basically the years from puberty to menopause, age 13 to 51 on average, or all of your fertile years

Perimenopause begins when your ovaries start to run out of eggs, and your fertility hormones slow down production; usually in mid 40s

Menopause is diagnosed when you haven't had a period for 12 months; the average age when this is diagnosed in UK is 51

Post menopause is the rest of your beautiful life, no longer hostage to hormone fluctuations

As I've said several times already, be prepared to notice the first symptoms of perimenopause during early to mid-forties. For some women these symptoms are mild and for others some of them are noticeable but manageable. For other women some are life limiting and will lead to decisions such as giving up their working life or their romantic partner. If you prepare well now, you give yourself the best chance of gliding gracefully through a gentle menopause.

Age 45 and over you don't need a blood test to confirm perimenopause, age and symptoms are enough to be offered hormonal support. Younger than 45 with irregular periods and peri symptoms may need investigation for potential POI (premature ovarian insufficiency) go and talk to your doctor.

There are some remedies I've heard about which seem to offer more support to more women than others. Suggestions are - drinking half a pint of soymilk daily, taking a quality calcium supplement, and daily magnesium supplement. Be careful however, because you don't need to supplement calcium if you have dairy in your diet.

If you enjoy alcohol, I know how easy it is to open a bottle of wine when the day's been tough, I did it, all my colleagues did too. Around menopause time, you don't need those empty calories, alcohol disrupts sleep and it can trigger hot flushes and night sweats.

Your life might be full and busy but fitting in exercise is as important as a good eating pattern. Health is wealth, not a large bank account. At this middle stage of life, you are setting yourself up for the next 50 years, so make them lean, fit and contented, then you'll have choices instead of crutches.

In your mid 40s, earliest symptoms you should expect are: -

- Irregular periods, sometimes very heavy, sometimes non-existent
- Hot flushes during the day and night sweats
- Emotional upheaval; tearful, angry, sad, overwhelmed, hopelessness

In your later 40s: -

- All of the above, plus
- Loss of personal confidence and drive to get things done
- Loss of immediate recall of names and facts

- Anxiety over the smallest of tasks and decisions
- Lack of focus and concentration
- Joint pain, especially spine, hip, knees
- Worsening sleep disturbances
- Hair thinning
- Weight gain around the midriff.

I know many women in their forties who have young children and elderly parents, who work full time themselves. It's a great deal to manage, as well as their own household. How will life change as your perimenopause begins?

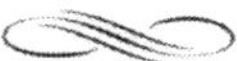

50's freedom, finally free of sanitary supplies, maybe.

Twelve months without a period means you are now past perimenopause, have gone through menopause and are now post-menopausal. Great, is that it then? No, sorry you're just getting warmed up.

Lots of women I know experienced only mild symptoms in their peri menopause; but just when they thought it had all passed them by, they had a jolt when symptoms became a problem. Don't be complacent and ignore problems, especially bladder, emotional and sexual.

Early post-menopause: -

- All of the above experienced in your 40's, plus
- Brain fog, poor decision making, memory loss – this all continues
- Personal confidence can take a nosedive
- Skin becomes drier and needs more moisturising

- Hair becomes drier and of course your colour needs attention more often (if you colour it)
- Urinary incontinence could become a problem, a little leakage at first, getting worse in time
- Urinary infections can be a recurrent problem
- Dry and sore vagina, no matter how much stimulation, it just isn't moist and welcoming
- Occasionally vague 'fishy' odour from a discoloured vaginal discharge
- Vaginal prolapse is common, (urge to pee more often and wanting to 'bear down' are signs of this)
- Bloating and weight gain, your midriff may join forces with belly
- Overflowing bra cups
- Facial wrinkles deepen and complexion changes, developing dark freckles anywhere
- Eyebrows go rogue and whiskers appear randomly around chin and mouth
- Vision gets poorer and most women need magnifying spectacles at least
- You could possibly be troubled by heart palpitations and pains in your chest
- Pains in chest that feel like a heart attack but are often dreadful indigestion
- Back pain is a common complaint and potential bone fractures from late 50s

All the above are common symptoms in females who don't supplement their oestrogen. Those who do find a supplement which works for them will usually experience fewer and milder symptoms.

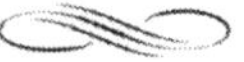

60s sashay into the sunset - the really great news is that almost all of the earlier symptoms disappear as your body has become re-balanced and is getting on without fertility hormones. However, the long-term effects of loss of oestrogen can create problems: -

- Hot flushes and night sweats reduce and by mid 60s are infrequent if felt at all

- If urinary problems have developed, they will be worse, so do your exercises (see chapter on bladder), moisturise your vulva often, and discuss a topical vaginal oestrogen supplement with your healthcare specialist
- Vaginal imbalance should be resolved but vaginal dryness and thinning of skin might be worse – see above
- Your bones lose density rapidly and bone fractures, especially wrist, are common
- Wrinkles and frown lines deepen and join up
- Whiskers, and their removal, needs constant vigilance
- There may be a need to re-adjust your mindset, having become used to the 'brain fog' of midlife, it's too easy to assume that is normal – it's not
- Heart disease is life limiting in the extreme; so prevention takes the form of good diet and regular exercise that makes you breathe faster for more than ten minutes

Long term health issues - once your body stops producing oestrogen, you are at greater risk of developing osteoporosis, heart disease, and Alzheimer's. In fact, 1 in 2 deaths in post-menopausal women in America is from heart disease.

Compare that with 1 in 29 deaths in post-menopausal women being from breast cancer. Women focus on the thought that oestrogen causes breast cancer, and completely ignore how much protection oestrogen will give their heart.

So, what can you do to support your body and protect it from these later life stage diseases?

Of course, the answer is similar to the one asked about menopause symptoms; everyone's menopause is different, and every single body reacts differently to nutrition, exercise and medication.

Here are some ideas: -

- Entering your mid-forties with good nutrition and a light body weight is optimum for having the easiest, least disruptive menopause.

- Exercise of some kind every day is good for your mental and physical health and also helps to prevent joint and muscle pains. You'll find sleep is better after exercise too. Get family involved and exercise is even better
- Exercise which causes the long bones in your legs to have impact (think jogging, bouncing, dancing, walking moderately fast) is very helpful to maintain excellent bone health everywhere in your body
- Whatever you eat in whatever portions, (I include health supplements of all kinds) can never equal what your body used to produce, nor give you the same amount of oestrogen and progesterone as can hormone supplement therapy
- Many women who have been thin all of their lives due to diet, develop symptoms of osteoporosis in their 60's. You need to have calcium in your diet daily as well as vit D3, so get a proper supplement or learn how to get it from nutrition and don't ignore the importance of it. Osteoporosis is dreadful and avoidable in the 21st century.
- Be realistic about the weight you expect to lose while going through your menopause. Limit the damage caused by overeating and drinking wine daily by having smaller portions and choosing something non-alcoholic before dinner.

If you understand the risks and are prepared to do the work required, by the time you are late 50's and in your 60's you will emerge as a fit and strong woman with at least another thirty years of healthy and joyful life ahead.

Now you can draw breath and re-evaluate your life in the light of your post-menopausal state.

In the UK there has been an enormous shift in the number of people discussing menopause over the last year, remedies and symptoms are all over TV and media; this is fabulous and has opened up a wider conversation about older women in the workplace. In the UK we now have to wait until age 65 to claim our Government Pension and many women have to work until then. If you have to earn income until 65 it's even more important to look after yourself and stay strong, fit and healthy. That habit begins in your younger years as you prepare for menopause, and as long as you can walk, you can take exercise.

Continue to moisturise your vagina in the same way you do your face and neck with paraben free and safe products such as 'Sylk', 'Yes Yes' etc. (instructions on the box). You can thank me later. Or, if you already suffer bladder infections, vaginal discharge, or painful intercourse, go and ask your doctor for 'Vagifem' or similar, which is a vaginal preparation containing low-dose oestrogen and is designed to re-build the thinning skin and stop those problems recurring.

And, sail away.

BLADDER INCONTINENCE

ONE OF THE MOST COMMON SYMPTOMS of ageing, and this is possibly the most embarrassing, and least discussed. Around 30% of 30-39-year-old women will develop some degree of bladder incontinence; 55% of 80-90-year olds, and among residents in nursing homes, 65% have bladder incontinence. We rarely discuss it and I think that's because the word incontinence brings images of the frail and elderly or the very sick with their bedpans.

I had a friend who sold a pharmaceutical product designed to take care of this problem, but my colleague described the type of patient who would benefit from her product as "the old lady with pissey knickers" which offended me at the time. The word *incontinence* certainly doesn't bring into mind an image of a vital and energetic woman, rushing through her life with a list of fifty things to do, a working day to get through and a family to feed and nurture. If you develop either type of bladder incontinence you have a choice of pad up and put up, do your pelvic floor exercises for the rest of your life or, see your doctor for a non-systemic treatment which has a high rate of success in resolving the issue.

If you know the comedian Billy Connolly and are a fan, then you might have watched a sketch he did some years ago about a new invention called 'incontinence pants' which he demonstrated on stage, creating total hysteria in his audience. You can find it on 'you-tube' during one of his very best stage shows called 'an audience with Billy

Connolly'. Funny in the extreme, but I'm sure that some of his audience were suffering leakage while they were laughing.

Let me tell you my experience of bladder problems, even though I truly don't want to, because you need to understand this. The best advice I ever got from anyone who understands this issue is that you must exercise your pelvic floor every day and keep it toned up. This advice comes from written articles as well as health care professionals. Well, I taught Pilates exercise classes for several years between the ages of 39-45, and for six years before that I taught aerobics, so my pelvic floor should have been tight as a drum. Hmmm, it was tight during childbirth but not so much during menopause.

Before you get too worried, I have to add that my story isn't true of every woman, and many women get through menopause with only vague symptoms of bladder incontinence.

I was invited to a midsummer fancy-dress party which was a wonderful outdoor barbeque with many friends present. A DJ was playing great tunes and I was on the dance floor; not many moves into the dance I felt my bladder relax and very quickly my white linen trousers were soaked.

I carried on dancing, hoping that my dance partner wouldn't notice the aroma of fresh urine, in the same way that when I wore pads in my knickers as a schoolgirl, I hoped the boys wouldn't notice that aroma. Clearly no one did because not a word was said (or perhaps the other guests were just too polite or confused by the unexpected). I was shocked and distressed but luckily had drunk enough wine that I could carry on as though nothing had happened, nothing to see here.

By far the most dreadful experience was while I was at work. The entire company was staying in a beautiful castle on a huge estate and our 'black tie' celebration event was beyond lavish. Some of my team were in their twenties and after dinner they ordered 'shots'. Just because I was in my fifties wasn't a reason to say no, so I drank one and continued to enjoy the party. However, when I stood to leave the table and take myself off to bed, my bladder malfunctioned. I was wearing a very lovely black velvet dress and expensive shoes, and at the beginning of the evening had felt vibrant and attractive. The long walk back to my room, along endless corridors was just me, alone, dribbling into my lovely shoes the entire way. I arrived back in my bedroom, stripped off my expensive dress, took a shower and cried very hard for a long time.

I finally realised that ***alcohol played a large part*** in all of those incidents and understood that the reason my bladder couldn't hold its contents was because alcohol relaxes muscles, and the bladder is just a muscle. Alcohol wasn't the only reason though, and as years went by, I began to leak just as I was walking around the house, walking my dog or grocery shopping.

Girlfriends tell me they sometimes don't make it to the bathroom if they wake up needing a pee, meaning soggy pjs, bedsheets or slippers! There's a phrase 'door key incontinence' which is used among health care professionals; and it's used to describe the moment you put the key into your front door and desperately need a wee. Alternately, just as you're locking the door, having been to the toilet already, you feel the need to go again, just in case you can't make it to the next toilet. When I still couldn't resolve the problem through exercise, I thought it just wasn't going to get better and I needed to wear panty liners forever. What I felt was a kind of numb acceptance that I was unlikely ever again to go dancing or to the gym or jog around the village because I was always wet.

The knock-on effect of this was that I felt grubby all the time, and occasionally disgusted by the problem, so I reduced my daily fluid intake to a minimum in an attempt to stop the leakage because I was working full time.

The problem is that drinking only a minimum of water every day causes physical and mental dehydration resulting in a stressed body and regular headaches, brain fog and poor decision making. Do those symptoms sound familiar? They do because they're symptoms of the peri menopause and I need you to see that it's easy to fall into a vicious cycle of cause and effect when it comes to self-management.

Something else I'd like you to understand is that at no point did I think my weak bladder was caused by my peri menopause or that I could do anything about it, apart from more of the same exercises. More importantly, at no time did any of the health professionals I saw tell me that the problem might be caused by hormones.

If they had I might have known that I could maybe do something to resolve it, along with exercises. I believed it was a problem that I needed to pad-up-and-put-up with, so I joined the tribe of middle-aged women with sanitary pads in my shopping basket.

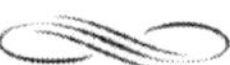

Eventually, I was sick of denying myself the life I used to have and went back to my doctor. I begged her for help in getting my life back, and I'm grateful that she referred me to a Consultant Urologist for tests.

The Urologist was a highly qualified and respected doctor, with many years of treating middle aged women, but not even he suggested that the problem could be caused by hormone shortage, nor did he discuss menopause. He did, however, offer me a new procedure which he was pioneering in the UK. This involved surgery to insert a kind of 'sling' made of mesh which would support my urethra. This would prevent leakage until I was able to deliberately relax my bladder and pass urine when I wanted to. Do you think I said no thanks? Hell no. I almost fell to the floor and kissed his feet when he said I was a good patient for the procedure.

All Urologists (bladder specialists) agree that a common bladder irritant is caffeine. Whether you take it in tea, coffee, energy drinks, soft fizzy drinks, or cold remedies, it will irritate your bladder and trigger a need to pass urine. If you have a hot drink at night, it's far better for your sleep quality to have hot chocolate or another milky drink. If you are feeling the need to go the toilet more often than you can improve the problem by drinking less caffeine.

What does happen to the bladder to cause this unwanted leakage?

The bladder is a muscle which expands like a balloon as it collects and holds urine. Your urine flows in an almost constant dribble from the kidneys into the bladder where it collects, and when your bladder feels full and you decide to empty it, the urine flows from the bladder out of your body through the urethra.

The urethra is usually supported and held closed by a 'sling' of muscle called your pelvic floor, which is attached to your pelvis at the front and back to support your pelvic organs and womb. There are two types of bladder incontinence which are described below.

The reason why bladder incontinence can be a symptom of the peri and menopause is because your oestrogen levels have dropped, and this causes the acidity to change within your vaginal area. It causes your pelvic muscles to weaken and the internal skin to become thinner, drier and more likely to become irritated. When your urethra is irritated then you may feel the need to pass urine more often. If the pelvic floor muscles are weaker, they may not be able to support your bladder and urethra as they used to, and leakage happens. Those of you who have given birth might remember that immediately prior to labour your pelvic muscles relax to allow the baby to pass through your cervix and out, same hormonal thing.

During perimenopause your periods will become irregular and you might find that your uterus swells up during the months when the lining doesn't shed. Your bladder sits in front of the uterus within your pelvis; therefore, your swollen uterus is likely to put pressure on your bladder which causes leakage.

Urinary infection can be caused by low levels of oestrogen. This feels and smells like cystitis, but your doctor can give you a better remedy than he would for cystitis. Don't just put up with it because it doesn't get better by itself, and once you have the problem resolved, you'll wonder what took you so long to manage it more actively. A prescription for Vagifem or Ovestin should help, since both claim to treat 95% of this type of recurring infection within two weeks.

Stress Incontinence is the term used for accidental leakage of urine when you cough, sneeze, run, jump, dance, or do anything physical that puts pressure on your bladder. This is a real problem because you might be put off doing the exact things which will reduce your chance of developing osteoporosis in later life, since anything like running, dancing, trampolining, etc are the best type of exercises to prevent it.

The muscles supporting the bladder can become damaged or weakened after childbirth. This type of incontinence is very common and in women over 40 years old, around 20% or one in five women will experience it. To improve bladder control you could exercise your pelvic floor very regularly from the age of 40, although it's never too late to begin, and the set of Kegel exercises and stopping the flow of urine while emptying your bladder (described below) are helpful.

Exercise alone can't make an immediate difference though because it may take several weeks of regular repetition before your muscles respond and tone up, and you must continue for ever. If exercise doesn't help enough, then your doctor can offer surgery, (as I describe above although other types of surgery can be offered) or low dose oestrogen (yam or soy) and you can choose from several applications.

Urge Incontinence is the term used for that feeling of having a full bladder and needing to empty it, but your brain doesn't get enough warning of this before the bladder empties itself. It may be a trickle or a flood. As a rough guide, if you're aged less than 40, this type of problem is possibly caused by a bladder infection or thinning of the tissues that make up the urethra, or even damage to the nerves which control the bladder. If you're over 40 it can also be caused by a lack of oestrogen which will affect the lining of your bladder and urethra.

Some women I spoke to reported regular dreams of sitting on the toilet to pass urine, only to wake up and realise they had wet pyjamas, this is called nocturia and I'm guessing that having to change your bed sheet in the middle of the night is a total passion killer. Again, this type of incontinence is very common, and many women have a combination of both stress and urge incontinence.

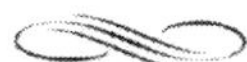

I urge you to take action if you suffer from either type of bladder incontinence or even a combination of both, as I did.

This symptom will not just go away post menopause, as emotional symptoms will, and actually will get worse with age. In the UK, at least 35% of women have avoided a situation that makes them laugh because of bladder weakness, that's a lot of joy to deny ourselves.

I've already said that alcohol makes incontinence worse and so does caffeine from tea and coffee, whereas drinking more plain water helps to keep your bladder clean and healthy. I've listed several websites (Resource section) where you can get more advice for bladder problems.

To support the bladder muscle a really helpful exercise is: when you're sitting on the toilet relax your muscles so that urine is flowing well, then tighten up your pelvic floor and stop the flow, hold the contraction for a count of ten, then release the flow and repeat. If you do this regularly it will help, as well as the Kegel exercises which are very similar to the type of prep you would do to strengthen your core lower abdominal muscles during Pilates and can involve a small machine.

The aim of low dose vaginal oestrogen is to relieve the symptoms of bladder incontinence, mainly the skin changes that take place in the tube from the bladder (urethra). These changes may result in symptoms of urinary frequency or urgency and discomfort passing urine. You may also be more prone to urinary tract infections. Local intravaginal oestrogen can help to relieve these symptoms.

Applying oestrogen via vaginal pessaries, or a donut kind of thing infused with oestrogen, or a gel applied externally, are all very successful in relieving this symptom. The oestrogen supplied in this way will improve the quality of the skin by normalizing its acidity and making it thicker and better lubricated.

The advantage of using local therapy rather than systemic therapy (i.e. hormone tablets or patches, etc.) is that much lower doses of hormone can be used to achieve good effects in the vagina, while minimizing effects on other organs such as the breast or uterus.

If you have had breast cancer and have persistent troublesome symptoms which aren't improving with vaginal moisturizers and lubricants, local oestrogen treatment may be a possibility. Your Urogynecologist will coordinate the use of vaginal oestrogen with your Oncologist. Studies so far have not shown an increased risk of cancer recurrence in women using vaginal oestrogen who are undergoing treatment of breast cancer or those with history of breast cancer.

You may also find vaginal oestrogen useful if you take hormone therapy at a low dose, still get bladder problems, but don't want to increase the dose of HRT. Just add in the vaginal oestrogen.

Your doctor might suggest you take a medication which calms the bladder down if it's overactive, but this type of med is called an anticholinergic, and is likely to dry out other areas you would like to stay moist. For example, your mouth, nose and eyes.

So, don't just continue buying sanitary pads and panty liners, go do something better and get on with your life.

The end of my story is that my bladder problems are relieved! I can jump and run, stay fit and energetic all day long without any leakage. I got my life back.

BONES, MUSCLES & JOINTS

Menopause is around the time when you might notice that every time you bend down to pick something up, there's a sound, a little like 'ooof' and it's coming from you. Once you catch yourself making this sound you should just laugh, most of us make it and it isn't a sign of old age, it's just a thing.

Joint pain isn't so amusing though, and many of you may begin to feel as though you slept on a rock as you make your way to the bathroom first thing in the morning. It can make the difference between anticipating your chosen exercise class or avoiding it, although going and enjoying the feeling of satisfaction at the end is always the best choice. When you notice joint pain and muscle ache, along with a change in your periods (if you have them), and begin feeling as though someone removed your temperature control, it's all the same problem. Production of oestrogen is slowing down and that will affect the elasticity of the cartilage and tendons which hold your bones together, hence the joint ache. Muscles feel stiffer too for the same reason and you could find that cramp is a problem.

YES, you are in perimenopause, NO you're not old.

Swimming or yoga is the best choice of exercise if you have a lot of pain as it obviously avoids putting pressure on the problem areas. As a friend said

"I tried yoga first time yesterday. I decided I had to do something as my joints and hips have been feeling really stiff. I would really recommend it because I woke up this morning for the first time in a long while feeling like my old self"

Another friend suggested this recipe: - "turmeric milk to ease joints. I make my own golden paste then mix a teaspoon into a cup of warm milk. A glug of local honey and drink it morning and night. Golden paste recipe is 1cup turmeric powder. 2cups water heated slowly stirring all the time. Simmer very gently for a few mins then remove from heat. Stir in tablespoon of coconut oil add 1 heaped teaspoon of black pepper and decant into jars. Will keep in the fridge for 2 weeks"

If you have concerns and are worried that the problem is more than lack of oestrogen, then have a conversation with your doctor. Osteoarthritis and rheumatoid arthritis are very different problems and it's possible that some of your family have either or both of them. If they have, then you may have some genes which make you likely to develop it as well.

Clearly, being overweight and/or obese will cause you much greater problems structurally. Obesity is an epidemic in the western world as I write this, and the disability industry is having a lot of fun creating huge profits for itself by supplying walking sticks and mobility aids to the population. Type 2 diabetes may not sound as much of a problem as Type 1, but I promise you it is actually worse and a great deal more difficult to treat. Especially if you smoke and/or drink alcohol regularly. Losing weight is the number one treatment to prevent type 2 diabetes.

Osteoporosis: the first sign that you may have developed osteoporosis is most likely to be when you have a fall or trip which results in a fracture of one of your long, thin bones. Wrist fractures are most common, spinal fractures less so. If you suffer a simple fracture over the age of 35, you are likely to be invited to have your bones screened or tested.

Simple bone screening is done by an ultrasound machine that measure the bone density in one heel. If low bone density is seen, you will be invited back for a scan with a DEXA machine.

- DEXA is a scan and is usually performed before a doctor prescribes medications for osteo to rebuild bone mineral density. The test is a special X-ray film taken of the hip and of the lower bones in the spine. The scan is repeated in one and a half to two years to measure response to treatment

What the doctor is measuring is your loss of bone density, or osteoporosis. The DEXA scan can calculate bone mineral density and compare it to the average of a healthy young woman. The World Health Organization defines osteoporosis as more than 2.5 standard deviations below that average rule. A condition known as osteopenia is where you have less severe bone loss of 1 to 2.5 standard deviations below the average rule.

The medications available for loss of bone density are all unpleasant and distasteful and many women need a reminder from their doctor to use it. You may need to stay on it for around 5 years; with a 'holiday' from treatment and further assessment to decide whether or not you go back onto it.

Prevent osteoporosis: two main things are very helpful in prevention, because that's what you should be aiming for. First is diet and second is exercise. The right time to begin prevention is now or yesterday

- Your diet needs to contain regular servings of some or all of these: oily fish, eggs, lamb's liver, calcium. All contain vitamin D which is vital for great bone health. Sunlight is free and available for some of the year all over the world, when it isn't a supplement can be taken which provides a minimum of 10mg daily. Calcium is necessary to help the body absorb vitamin D and that's available in many foods and supplements.
- Any exercise which puts strain on your long bones and joints is good. Many menopause symptoms can be relieved through exercise, the trouble is those symptoms leave you feeling that you just can't be bothered and the thought of going out and exercising is not high on your daily plan. If you're reading this book, I'm guessing that you already take reasonable care of yourself and have some type of favourite exercise. A recent study at the University of Leeds discovered that any exercise which puts strain on your joints is successful at reducing loss of

bone density. So that's jogging, dancing, brisk walking, bouncing on a trampoline, playing squash or tennis, etc. Team games or gym membership provide much more mental health support as well as fitness.

Please go to the Royal Osteoporosis Society for much more information. Web address in Resources.

DIGESTIVE CHANGES

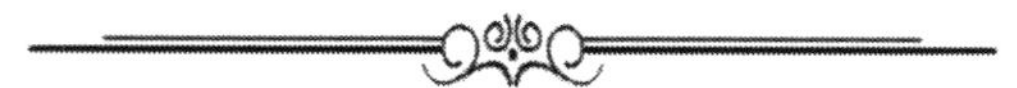

As discussed, oestrogen helps to maintain a healthy digestive system and it stands to reason that a shortage of it will cause changes within the system. We often experience abdominal pain, bloat, constipation and diarrhoea around the time of our periods, and this continues through perimenopause and beyond.

This symptom is usually what causes us to develop, almost overnight, a tummy which is full and often hard and painful. The first sign of bloat is the ever-tighter waistband and a need to pass wind. In fact, although it can be embarrassing in public, finding a quiet place to pass wind is a secret art of menopausal women.

How to defeat excess gas in your digestive system - there are a few things you can try to help with this symptom, most of them don't come from the doctor.

- Reduce the amount of animal protein eaten; meat has a habit of moving slowly through your intestines and creates a 'back-log' of other food which begins to ferment and make gas.

- Drink plenty of water; you should be drinking 2 litres of plain water daily for the best health. There are so many 'urban myths' about water – when to drink it and when not to drink it, whether tea and coffee are just as good, if it's carbonated or not -that it's difficult to know what to believe, but I promise you that drinking a lot of water all through the day and evening is a very good thing.
- *At first you will need to pee more, but then your body gets used to the quantity of water, every cell in your body becomes better hydrated, and your need to pee reduces. You probably wake in the night for a comfort break anyway. A good habit is to have a bottle full of fresh water in your car every day, or on your desk. Don't keep buying single use bottles from the garage or supermarket, you can buy reusable bottles in many shapes and sizes which are filled for free from your tap. I have a filter on my cold-water tap, and I fill jugs which chill in my fridge. The water is delicious, and my dogs love the taste too.*
- Stop drinking anything fizzy which is a whole bloat story by itself. If you really must, the exception will be champagne and prosecco, only because you're unlikely to be drinking that every day, all day (?) and it does have some medicinal power when drunk in moderation and in company. Any fizzy drink will dehydrate, which is another good reason to limit their use.
- Certain vitamins and minerals can help – magnesium is important for every cell in your body, and supports your digestive system, and Vitamin D is also really helpful. You can get magnesium from leafy veg such as spinach, whole grains, bananas, peanuts, figs and avocados etc.
- Eat more fibre which will speed up the passage of food along your intestines and bowel, and that will prevent food from getting stuck and fermenting, which creates gas. I have a green smoothie almost every day, (recipe in back of book) either for lunch or dinner and always eat porridge oats for breakfast, not the instant type which are too processed for me, but the big chunky (Americans call them 'steel cut') flakes of organic crushed oats. I eat my porridge with local honey, cinnamon and frozen raspberries, altogether it's a feast.
- Reduce your stress levels because stress can cause that dreadful fluttering in the pit of your stomach, which often translates into disturbed digestion. Cortisol is the culprit of this, and it will slow down your digestive system. So, instead of reaching for a snack based on sugar, learn how to breathe deeply and use that to satisfy

your need to relax. Also, avoiding anything which is based on yeast; beer, lager, wine, bread, which will feed the gas inside of you.

Find a delicious herbal tea which isn't sweetened and drink that instead of some hot drinks with milk. I have a favourite which is liquorice and peppermint, enough to satisfy my cravings for sweetness but almost zero calories and really good for my digestion.

Discover how your body reacts to food by paying attention and keeping a diary of what caused your tummy to bulge and what didn't. Try to eliminate all of those foods and drinks that did, and then re-introduce them one by one until your diet is acceptable.

Look, I know this is more difficult when you have a partner or family to feed, but it seems to me that most families have a staccato way of eating which feeds different elements of the family when they need to be fed; the trick for you is to not eat every time a member of your family is being fed! Many families discover that having one or two meals per week when they all sit down together is a fabulous way to maintain cohesion in busy lives and is successful at maintaining a strong family dialogue and dynamic where every individual is paid attention to and heard.

HAIR LOSS/INCREASE

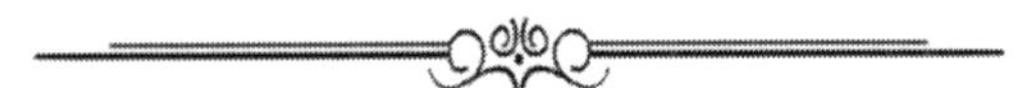

HAIR LOSS and changes in the quality, colour and texture of your hair happens to almost every woman during perimenopause and continues during menopause. It happens because your body slows the production of oestrogen which is important in the growth and health of your hair, so it looks thinner and you will possibly notice more hair in the plughole. It's just another reason why a lot of women feel 'less' everything – feminine, attractive, vibrant, youthful, useful – and there is no right or wrong way to deal with it.

There are several shampoos and health supplements which may be helpful in reducing the amount of hair loss and stimulating new hair growth. They can be found in supermarkets as well as health food stores.

Hair loses its colour as we age, and many men and women notice their first grey hairs during their twenties, as I did, so this isn't a result of menopause. The hair follicle produces colour pigment and its ability to produce colour reduces over time. Each hair follicle will produce a new hair every two to three years and eventually, the new hair will be colourless so that it will look white or grey.

Many women never colour their hair and allow the grey to gradually take over their natural colour. Some women choose to cut it all off and stop colouring it. Other women decide to continue colouring their hair until they die! It's a choice, no right or wrong, and the best thing is that any of us can change our hair at any time we want to.

When I first noticed changes in my hair, I already wore it short and because most of my hair turned grey in my late thirties, I always had a full colour of blond. As the dark roots turned grey, I changed my full head colour to having highlights which blended the blond and grey and was very successful at not showing root growth. From around the age of 50 I grew my hair long and kept it long until my mid-sixties. Last year I cut it short again and this year I decided to stop having it coloured at all, so I now have short silver hair, and it's very much admired by younger women. Luckily, this colour is having a trend at present, so my white hair doesn't so much look like a little old lady, as an on-trend statement! Lucky me, I'm saving a fortune and very happy about that.

The opposite problem of hair loss from the top of your head is having extra and new hair growth on your face. Billy Connolly. again, said something along the lines of, presuming mother nature knows what she's doing, could anyone explain why I now need longer, darker hair in my nose and ears

Occasionally I notice hair growing along a friend's top lip, and sometimes it isn't just a pale moustache but bristly. Years ago, I entered into a sacred pact with my two best friends that when we were together, we would look at each other critically, and when a rogue bristle or dark hair was noticed we would mention it. We never go so far as to pluck at each other as a monkey might, but it's been a great comfort to know someone who loves me is supporting me in this area.

It only works when we're wearing our specs of course. I also keep tweezers beside a magnifying mirror which sits in good morning light and check myself often. My eyesight isn't so good these days and things are a bit 'soft focussed' so chin hair isn't so easy to see. If you don't want to pluck out these hairs with tweezers there are several other methods of hair removal and, by now, you'll be familiar with most of them. When it comes to thicker or darker hair growth on your arms and legs, plucking with tweezers won't work so well. Make your choice from salon treatments such as waxing, threading, laser removal with IPL (intense pulsed light) or electrolysis; and using depilatory creams at home are several solutions.

Finally, even though this isn't part of the above conversation, nipple hair is very common – just sayin.

HEADACHE AND MIGRAINE

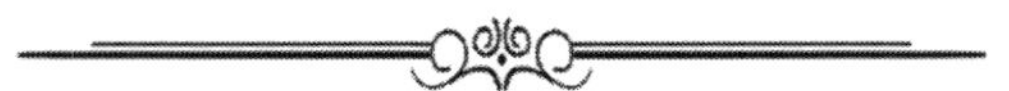

THERE'S GOOD NEWS and bad news around perimenopause, menopause and headache or migraine. Which would you like first?

If you regularly get a headache around your period, then these might be more frequent and worse during perimenopause. However, once you are past menopause and your hormones have regulated themselves, you should find your hormonal headaches stop.

There are some women who never experienced headache or migraine around their period who START to suffer migraine post menopause. I was one of those and endured countless difficult half-hours while my eyes developed the visual disturbance called a 'migraine aura'. I must have had several of these events before I actually paid attention to them, or perhaps they just became more severe over a short period of time.

What happens to me is that I notice a 'chink' or a disturbance in the outer corner of one of my eyes, usually the right one. Then this develops until my vision is like looking through a kaleidoscope. (I hope that makes sense). That effect then spreads over to the other eye and after around a half hour my vision returns to normal.

I rarely get a headache afterwards and only occasionally have felt a bit sick. I've noticed one trigger which is bright sunlight – but I live in the Lake District part of the UK, so unexpected bright sunlight doesn't happen too often.

If you choose to take a prescription for hormone therapy and find that your headaches or migraines are worse, talk to your Doctor about it and you may find that changing your oestrogen therapy from a pill to patch is helpful, because they are proven to be less likely to trigger the problem than oestrogen in a pill.

What you eat can have an impact on headaches. If you notice your headaches or migraines happening more often, try to keep a diary of what you ate before the event, just to see if you can figure out what your 'trigger' is. Common dietary triggers include alcohol, especially red wine, aged cheeses like Parmesan, caffeine, chocolate, dairy products.

Taking exercise is also good for prevention of headaches. If you are able, a walk outside in nature is easy, even in the city. Experts suggest taking 30 minutes of exercise three or four times a week is good. If you enjoy using the gym then do that, spinning in a cycling class, swimming, team sports, lots of choices.

Remember to warm up before activities because preparing your body for exercise can prevent a headache.

Acupuncture is an alternative medicine which uses needles to stimulate the body's energy pathways. It's a traditional Chinese medicine and is well documented as helpful in many systems of the body.

Relaxation therapy can be helpful. Learning how to be mindful or aware of the way your body responds to stress and muscle tension is a way of reducing the level of pain during an event.

Cognitive behavioural therapy is often used, along with relaxation techniques, for stress relief and pain management.

Water intake is also crucially important for reducing headache events. When the body is dehydrated a headache is often the first sign. If you have regular night sweats or hot flushes through the day, it's likely that you'll be short of minerals as well, to replace them, put a sachet of Dioralyte (or similar) into your water bottle every day. Try to always have water with you and take every opportunity to ask for water with a cup of tea or coffee. Many cafes now have a water station alongside the cutlery.

Vitamins and minerals supplements are often helpful, but always mention what you're taking when you discuss hormone therapy with your doctor. Suggested supplements are vitamins B2, D3, calcium, coenzymeQ10, and magnesium.

MENSTRUATION CHAOS

FIRST SIGN of oestrogen production slowing down will be when your periods are disrupted. You may notice a missed period, longer periods of bleeding, or flooding when you least expect to start bleeding, spotting at the wrong times; all horrid and disruptive in the worst possible way.

This is why menstruation is chaotic during perimenopause: -

- **Normal periods** happen around every 28 days, the cycle begins when the pituitary and hypothalamus glands secrete hormones which trigger the ripening of an egg in your ovaries
- After an egg is released or ovulated, progesterone is produced and works along with oestrogen to create all that's necessary for a foetus to grow inside your womb.
- If the egg is unfertilised the oestrogen and progesterone levels drop, and your womb discards its lining which creates menstruation
- **Perimenopause periods** begin when fewer of the remaining eggs ripen, and no eggs are ovulated from your ovaries
- When an egg is not released or ovulated, there is no creation of progesterone and oestrogen carries on creating a lining inside your womb during the first half of the month.
- Without progesterone to counteract the oestrogen, the lining is not released and becomes thicker; although you might notice some spotting of blood when you would have had a normal period.
- If this happens again next month and perhaps the next, the womb lining can be evicted suddenly and you have to deal with an excess

of blood, sometimes in clots, often at the most unexpected and inconvenient time

This can be quite a worry if you don't understand what's going on, especially if you've had thirty or so years of regular straightforward periods.

Around 25% of women get really heavy periods during their perimenopause, so, once you realise, you're in perimenopause, keep a diary and always be prepared when out of your home. Try using the 'double up' approach with both a tampon and a pad for heavy periods, if this is possible for you. You could also make sure that any sanitary machines at work contain products for heavy bleeds.

If you currently use a Mirena/Jaydess coil for contraception, you can continue with it until after your menopause, and will then need to have it removed. These coils contain progesterone which prevents the uterus from developing the lining required for a fertilised egg to grow into a foetus. However, the presence of progesterone offers no relief from menopausal symptoms, so you may realise you're in perimenopause only when you begin to notice hot flushes or night sweats, or other symptoms discussed within this chapter.

It's fairly common for a doctor to suggest the insertion of a coil to relieve heavy bleeding during the menopause.

The 'mini' contraceptive pill also contains only progesterone so offers no relief from menopausal symptoms. If you're on the 'mini' pill and notice any of the perimenopause symptoms are causing you problems, then you can switch to a combined contraceptive pill which will give you progesterone and oestrogen, and this will mask your symptoms fairly effectively. Or, you could add a low dose oestrogen patch or apply oestrogen gel. Again, all women are different and have different responses to medication, so this is your journey to find what works for you along with your doctor.

The average woman will go through the period called perimenopause for around four years, but for some it's six or seven, then periods will stop altogether. The months when you have no period are sometimes called the 'climacteric' or menopause transition. Once there has been no period for a full year if you are over 50, you are medically post menopause.

As for fertility, the rule is that you are still fertile until you've had one full year without a period if you're over 50, and if under 50 you need to have two full years without a period. Until those time frames are complete then you're considered to be still fertile and able to conceive, so if you don't want to, you need to have some form of contraception in use.

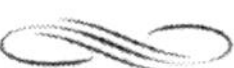

Surgical menopause is necessary for a number of reasons which can happen to a woman at any stage of life. For a woman to go into immediate menopause after surgery, both ovaries need to be removed because, even if a small part of one ovary is left, it can produce oestrogen.

A hysterectomy is a major operation for a woman which is only recommended if other treatment options have been unsuccessful, and if she has decided that she does not want to have any more children.

For full information around surgical menopause and hysterectomy, please go to https://www.nhs.uk/conditions/hysterectomy/why-its-done/ .

The most common reasons for having a hysterectomy are: -

- heavy periods – which can be caused by fibroids
- pain in the pelvic area – which may be caused by endometriosis, unsuccessfully treated pelvic inflammatory disease (PID), adenomyosis or fibroids
- prolapse of the uterus
- cancer of the womb, ovaries or cervix

Heavy periods are usually measured by the amount of blood lost during a period. Every woman is different in the amount of blood loss which she would USUALLY notice during a period. If you have always had heavy blood loss (as defined below), or if the amount of blood loss has changed recently, you need to have a conversation with your doctor.

A heavy period can be measured by these: -

- you need to change your sanitary products every hour or two
- you are passing blood clots larger than 2.5 cm (about the size of a 10p coin)
- you bleed through to your clothes or bedding
- you need to use 2 types of sanitary product together (for example, tampon and pad)

As well as the heavy loss of blood, some women also experience other symptoms, such as stomach cramps and pain. This pain can have a significant impact on quality of life.

Fibroids can grow and cause heavy periods, so it's important that you get yourself examined. Fibroids can make intercourse painful and can be the cause of urinary problems and constipation, so if you discover them early, the outcome will be better.

Pelvic pain can be caused by pelvic inflammatory disease (PID) which is a bacterial infection in the reproductive system. Again, see your doctor and have some treatment because the sooner this is resolved the better the outcome.

Endometriosis is caused when some of the cells which line the womb, escape via the fallopian tubes and inhabit other areas of the reproductive system. These cells can cause adhesions and scarring which causes pain and inflammation.

Adenomyosis is where the tissue that normally lines the womb starts to grow within the muscular walls of the womb. This can make your periods extra painful and can be the cause of pelvic pain.

Prolapse of the uterus happens when the tissues and ligaments that support the womb weaken, causing it to drop down from its normal position. This can cause back pain, leakage of urine caused by pressure on the bladder, and a feeling that something is dragging down inside your vagina and can make intercourse difficult.

CANCER of the cervix, ovaries, uterus or fallopian tubes, can also be reasons for a doctor to recommend a hysterectomy.

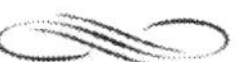

Making a decision to have a hysterectomy - if you have cancer, and your doctor recommends that a hysterectomy is the only treatment option, then you have little choice.

If you have other health problems which your doctor feels can be improved or cured by a hysterectomy, these are some questions you should ask yourself: -

- Are my symptoms seriously affecting my quality of life?
- Have I explored all other treatment options?
- Am I prepared for the possibility of an early menopause?
- Do I still want to have children?

Do not be afraid to ask your doctor as many questions as you want.

New exciting research is being done on the harvesting of healthy ovarian tissue from patients requiring this type of surgery. This could mean that for a woman in her 20 or 30s, she could possibly still become pregnant from her own eggs within her own harvested ovarian tissue. This work is still in early stages but offers hope to many women who have to surrender their ovaries because of breast cancer.

If you need to have both of your ovaries removed it will cause you to go immediately into menopause without passing through perimenopause. You should expect to be counselled and supported by your local Consultant Gynaecologist and advised on hormone therapy and alternatives. Your GP may not have enough expertise to support you adequately, so if this support is not available, you should ask for referral to a centre which can offer it.

Male doctors don't really understand the impact which menopause has on women and their families. Therefore, it has been known for a surgeon to advise his patient that he 'may as well take both ovaries, since menopause is not a big deal'. Do ask if it's necessary to remove both.

There are some other solutions for improvement of heavy bleeding during periods.

Prostap injections are used to reduce the thickness of the lining in the uterus and can be helpful when fibroids are present. Prostap is a hormone inhibitor and can be used prior to any of the ablation procedures, or to treat endometriosis and fibroids.

Ablation of the lining of the uterus is a non-surgical procedure which can be very helpful in reducing the amount of blood loss during a period, or, preventing blood loss in between periods. There are several methods of ablation available and these range from using cryoablation to microwave energy, radiofrequency to balloon therapy. All of these procedures require implements to be inserted into your uterus through your cervix via the vagina.

Only consider any of the ablation procedures if you have no interest in having more children.

For full information on all of these, please go to the NHS website mentioned above.

MENOPAUSE MIND

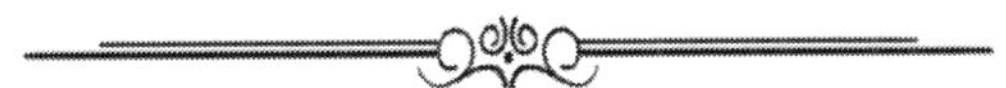

What is a C.R.A.F.T moment?

FEMALE EMOTIONS are controlled in large part by hormones from puberty until well after menopause, fact. Or about half of our lives. What our menfolk don't understand (not their fault) is that there are times when we can't control ourselves emotionally, just can't, and we sometimes/occasionally/regularly, (apparently) go crazy.

I have an ex-husband who would hear a particular tone in my voice, look at me, lift one corner of his mouth and speak those dreadful words "oh God, it's that time of the month isn't it". I know that you know what I'm describing when I say that red mist descended and I could turn into 'The Hulk' in a moment, no matter who else was in our company. I'm not suggesting that you make your husband an 'ex' but I hope that I can help you to help him understand what we women need from our men at these times.

It's called a loving embrace and has nothing to do with sensual touch or kissing or needing sex. What I always wanted/needed, and what women hope for, is the kind of hug that lasts for as long as I wanted it to without him thinking or feeling that it's going to lead to more intimate action. It might, but as soon as he thinks it will, you will feel his thought and feel emotionally unsafe and then the feelings of comfort can spiral into despair. If you go through pre-menstrual syndrome or PMS every month then it's more likely that you'll continue to have similar changes in mood while you go through peri and menopause.

During the peri and menopause, you'll continue to ride this rollercoaster of emotions, but in many cases, (sorry) it actually is worse than PMS – the peaks are higher, and the troughs are lower. The only good news is, now you know there's an end in sight for these emotional disturbances; and, unless you supplement with hormone therapy, the hormones will eventually re-balance once your menopause is stable (sometimes ten years). I compare this symptom and the affect it has on us with puberty, only in reverse.

Again, please let me make clear, just as not every woman gets PMS, not every woman will experience all of these distressing emotions or any of them, and not necessarily to the same degree.

For most women the menopause arrives at a time when their life is at a crossroads of change and renewal. Children may be in their own homes, at university or leading their own lives while still living at home. Your career will possibly be at its height and your need to perform to highest standards puts you under great stress. It might be a time when you and your husband are thinking about downsizing your home which is at best stressful. For many women who have their babies later in life, their children still need mothering, but their own parents now need more care, the typical 'sandwich' situation.

It has been noticed by many doctors who work in psychiatry and psychology, that not only do women more frequently report cognitive difficulties as they transition from pre menopause to perimenopause to post menopause; but they also perform more poorly on standardized neuropsychological tests. Particularly tests of verbal memory, aspects of executive function, and processing speed. Women often describe these deficits as 'brain fog', and they and their doctors may blame the sleep deprivation associated with hot flushes and night sweats.

While these common menopausal symptoms can add to the severity of memory problems, they are not the primary cause of cognitive issues in these women. Meaning that lack of sleep, while debilitating, is not the only reason why your ability to function at a high level is reduced as you go through menopause.

Here are a few comments from women struggling to manage their own emotional lives, I'm grateful for their openness and haven't altered any of them:

"I'm tired and having a real struggle this week with emotions, I've been teary and snappy and I cannot concentrate on my work even though I'm busy and need to get a document written this week... which I still haven't started, just keep looking at the screen. I'm fed up of bleeding and rowed with my partner last night so he's not talking to me today. No point to this really than to just put it out there, somewhere that people understand. I just want to snuggle back in bed and not get up until I feel more human again... whenever that may be! I'm not looking for sympathy, just need to hear someone to say they understand I suppose."

"I feel your pain!! I'm sat in Morrisons car park trying to get a grip! I feel tired, fat, niggly, cold, fed up, you name it I feel it today! I too just want to go home put on my pjs and lie on the sofa and watch crap tv and eat crusty bread and cheese followed by lots of cake and tea, instead I shall put a smile on my face and attempt to go and run my business and have salad for lunch, hang on in there, we can do this"

"So, the weather has changed quite dramatically. On my way to work yesterday it was sleeting and 2°C. Is anyone else still dressing for summer and risking freezing to death, so as to avoid boiling to death when a flush comes on? I don't think I'll ever wear sleeves again!"

"It's good to know that I'm not the only one going through some of the horrible symptoms, as I can very much so relate to nearly all of them. I'm trying my very hardest to try & keep off any medications for it, I've just come off Citalopram for anxiety (as I didn't think it was doing anything, but think I certainly need something at times). I've

been Menopausal since the age of about 48, I'm now 56, just how long do we have to put up with these symptoms, as they seem to be going worse & not better. Never knew it could completely change a person so much, feel like a different person...Angry/Sad/Emotional/Frightened/Panic attacks/no self-confidence/joint aches/pains/the list goes on"

*"My sister used to call her hot flushes, brain fog etc, her CRAFT moments. As in, can't remember a f*****g thing!"*

My own menopause coincided with the early stage of a new and challenging career, plus my son returned from university with health problems which needed a lot of care and attention. The day he arrived home I collected him from the train station, he went to bed and I took a call from a local hospital to say my mother (83) had fallen and dislocated her shoulder, could I go and collect her and take care of her. The only lightness of that day came from discovering Mum's story.

She had slipped on frosty ground while hanging out her laundry and hurt her shoulder. Knowing she had an appointment with the local undertaker later that morning, she pulled herself together and made ready, then the black car arrived to take her to the cemetery so that she could choose a plot for herself and my Dad's ashes. I began to laugh when, having completed business and finding a lovely spot on a hill, the undertaker asked if she wanted to be dropped off anywhere and she replied, "the hospital please". She was being interviewed by the A&E nurse who asked how Mum had arrived at the hospital and when Mum told her she arrived in a hearse, even the hospital staff were laughing. Poor Mum had to be in a sling for weeks, needing help to get dressed in the early days.

My son took almost 6 years to recover, but my new career somehow blossomed and provided us with a very good income and a pension. At the time I was deeply grateful to my brother and sister in law who re-located to my hometown for a couple of years and were able to support me during the worst of days. I guess we never know how life will unfold.

Irritability, moodiness and overwhelm. I know so many women who are shouting from the roof tops for understanding, crying into the wind/wine bottle for someone to help them. A woman can go from speaking in a loving tone to a child, then with a turn of her head, snarl with fury at someone else. This unpredictability is what men just cannot understand and when he closes down it makes a woman cry even harder.

Many women already feel they're no longer attractive, or they're invisible, they're worthless, and inadequate. When you feel that you're trying to do everything that's expected of you, and do it well, but still feel that you're getting it all wrong, it's no surprise that you might dissolve into tears of rage and despair.

For me this is like being scratched by nylon thread in your underwear, you keep trying to smooth it down, but suddenly and without warning, the thread pops out and scratches again. The simplest things would make me cry, maybe my dog wouldn't let me brush her, or I couldn't complete a task on my computer even though I'd done the same task the day before.

Panic attacks and breath-taking anxiety arrive without invitation and you might find yourself suddenly unable to remember how to get home; you might feel afraid that you're going to faint, or die, or have a heart attack. This is partly because the physical symptoms can arrive suddenly and without reason. You might notice that your heart starts pounding or beats very fast. Feeling faint, dizzy or lightheaded – a friend once described to me that she felt someone had cracked an egg on top of her head and it was running over her scalp. You might feel hot or very cold, sweating, shaking or feeling sick, without reason. Your legs may turn to jelly or begin to shake. Similar to actual heart attack, a panic attack might make you feel pain in your chest, difficulty breathing or choking; it might frighten you and the fear will increase the feelings

If you feel any of the above, then please look at the website for Mind in the UK which is a free resource, address is in the Resource chapter.

Depression is a sneaky, conniving malfunction of your normal 'operating system'. I mean your thought processes and the workings of your mind. It can creep up on you slowly but surely and by the time you realise that you have a problem, it has drained your desire to do

anything about it. If you wanted to give depression a cartoon character, then it might be called Eeyore the donkey from Winnie the Pooh.

I reckon that I've lived with, and struggled to stave off, depression since my middle twenties, and that's not uncommon. Within the general population of the UK at any moment in time, one person in every five (includes children) will be having some type of treatment for some kind of depressive episode.

The question is, was depression always and throughout history, a problem that humans dealt with, or was it invented in the 1960s when scientists developed mind changing medications? Is depression always caused by life events and the way we manage ourselves during those events, or can it be caused by things out of our control? Perhaps the character of Elsa from the movie Frozen is a good model for childhood trauma.

Poor thyroid function can change the way we manage our emotional response; I know it sounds crazy but there is strong evidence that lack of a hormone called thyroxin is linked with depression. So perhaps talking this through with your doctor would be helpful.

A lack of daylight can also be a problem for many people living in countries such as Great Britain where cloud covers the sky for much of the year. A recent study suggested that taking a good vitamin D3 tablet is helpful for improving vitality in body and mind. I found a product called AdCalD3 in the chemist which has a clinically proven combination of calcium and vitamin D3. This combination will also help to stave off osteoporosis and joint breakages such as the wrist.

Depression will affect around 40% of the UK population at some time during their lifetime, it might be mild or moderate or full blown 'let me end my life now' kind of depression. At any time in the UK approximately 25% of the population is living with depression. It can develop over a period of time and it truly can creep up on you and sneakily take over your life. You think that life is going well and one day you just can't be bothered with anything and nothing seems to matter. You begin to think that no one cares about you and that you don't even matter. Sleep becomes a problem, both getting to sleep and staying asleep. Appetite is reduced so that, if you live alone, you may not bother making a meal for yourself. When you think you don't matter, your self-esteem level drops and you begin to isolate yourself from friends, then family, and one day you can't remember cleaning your teeth or wanting to wash yourself.

Anger isn't a part of depression because frankly you don't have the interest to be angry about anything. Work becomes a problem because concentration is progressively poor and focus drifts away. Energy levels drop and there might be a feeling that if you don't matter and no-one cares about you then why should you look after yourself and what's the point of living.

It often appears after a trauma or difficult life change, when you've managed your stress levels so that you function well enough to get by for a sustained period of time. Then one day you stop needing to manage yourself and the stress situation has resolved. However, the levels of 'happy chemicals' are low because the cortisol production you needed to get through the situation has reduced your ability to produce enough of them. This is the zone when low mood deepens into depression and it can happen to anyone, no matter how capable and well organized they are.

This situation was seen all around the UK when there was a severe nation-wide outbreak of foot and mouth disease and thousands of healthy animals had to be slaughtered to stop it spreading. I know farmers who took huge pride in their breeding programmes in order to maintain the highest breed standards and gene pool; only to find their life's work, their most valuable animals, lying in a heap one day. Once the clean-up was completed many of those farmers were diagnosed with depression because they simply couldn't see a way forward.

It certainly happened to me when, after my second divorce and vile battle with my ex, I pulled myself together long enough to land a really great sales position which had immense prospects. You can read all about this time of my life in the chapter within Goddess Academy.

What I would like to say here is that while driving home during menopause, I regularly had to fight the urge to turn left and run away before turning right and going home. When I turned off the motorway,

I only had a ten-minute drive before reaching home, but I simply couldn't face whatever would be waiting for me. It was exactly like the days before my divorce when I would pull up outside our home and feel sick in my stomach because I didn't know what kind of mood my husband would be in or what he would find fault with that day. Above all, talk to someone you trust who won't judge you as being unable to cope, and certainly don't trust your problem to anyone who isn't empathetic.

It's quite likely you will feel some of these symptoms to a greater or lesser degree, but if you've never suffered any of them before, then it's more likely that your emotional turbulence is caused by hormone imbalance than by mental health issues.

Please be aware, if you go to your doctor *and begin your conversation with emotional turbulence, he/she is more likely to discuss depression and anxiety than be willing to discuss menopause. The reason is simply that doctors are primed to care for their patient's mental health but usually have low understanding of 'menopause mind'. If your doctor insists on offering you an anti-depressant and won't discuss menopause, then go and see a different doctor until you find one who understands female health.*

I've never met a strong person with an easy past.

MENOPAUSE VAGINA

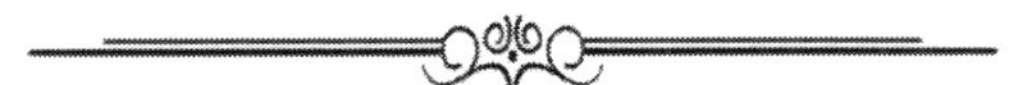

HERE'S the other least discussed but very common symptom within the long list of menopause symptoms. It isn't one of the first symptoms you'll notice but being prepared for it will help you. There's an obvious reason why women don't choose to discuss this with their friends or family, but not discussing it might leave you feeling that this problem is personal only to you.

Women often don't want to investigate because they fear it might be cancer. Or they might visit their doctor with complaints of itchy, discoloured and smelly (fishy) vaginal discharge, then find themselves in the unidentified infection clinic at the local hospital along with sexual health patients. That's not where you want or need to be.

The itching, soreness, discharge and dryness often begin after menopause. You might think you're through it when the doctor declares that you're post-menopausal, so the worst is over. It isn't. Some symptoms are less troublesome with the passing of years, and as your body becomes accustomed to the lack of oestrogen, many systems re tune themselves. Vaginal problems don't get better by themselves, however. In fact, global studies show that they get worse and can become chronic in older age. If you want to continue to live an energetic and vital life with dry panties and regular sex, pay attention here.

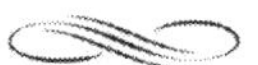

There are three main changes within the vagina caused by oestrogen reduction:

- First is that the pH. (acid/alkaline) levels within your vagina changes, therefore the bacteria within the vagina is out of balance. This causes the smell, the recurring infections, and the coloured discharge
- The second is the thinning and drying of the walls of the vaginal area. This can cause sex to be painful, feeling as though a cactus is inside your love tunnel. The lips of the vulva (called the labia) can become more sensitive, you might even feel that your labia rub painfully on underwear
- Also, loss of oestrogen can cause the muscles supporting your reproductive organs to lose power, and for some women a prolapse can happen. If you think that something no longer feels in the right place 'up there' go and talk to your doctor

I returned to riding a horse in the middle part of my menopause and found I was so uncomfortable I had to apply a thick sanitary pad to make it bearable. I even bought a pair of padded cycling shorts to wear beneath my jodhpurs. I had no idea that my sore vulva might be caused by menopause, just thought something out of my control had changed, and I never discussed it with my doctor. The itching and soreness did get better by itself, so I was a lucky one in this instance.

While going through the menopause your attitude towards general physical cleanliness may change. If you start to wash between your legs more often or change your soap/shower gel to a more perfumed one, it's possible that you'll disturb the already delicate balance of bacteria in your vagina. The answer is to wash with water, not soap, and don't be tempted to use a perfumed spray to keep yourself smelling fresh.

Vaginal Atrophy is the thinning, drying and inflammation of the vaginal walls and is usually caused by loss of oestrogen in the body.

Dyspareunia is recurrent or persistent pain associated with attempted or complete vaginal entry or penile vaginal intercourse. It can be felt at the entry to the vagina as well as higher up and is commonly felt around the cervix. While not assuming that all women have male partners, this pain can also be felt when vaginal entry is attempted with a finger, a tampon, or dildo.

In recent past the medical term which covers vaginal and urinary symptoms which are found during menopause has been changed to Genitourinary Syndrome of Menopause (GSM). Previously, the medical terms used were vulvovaginal atrophy and atrophic vaginitis.

This has been changed because those two phrases used by doctors did not adequately describe the full spectrum of symptoms and did not imply that the symptoms could be related to a reduction in oestrogen within women of menopausal age.

Indeed, very few women realise that these particular symptoms are a part of their menopause and are caused by hormones. Women would normally attribute them to ageing, so Gynaecologists rarely report women spontaneously consulting about these symptoms.

GSM now covers the terms vulvovaginal symptoms and lower urinary tract symptoms. These symptoms can considerably diminish Quality of Life (QOL) for postmenopausal women, therefore it's appropriate that better conversations are begun between doctor and patient to inform and educate on potential therapy.

Unlike vasomotor symptoms such as hot flushes and night sweats, GSM symptoms will not improve as the body re-balances its hormones, and for many women, they worsen. They can be chronic and although not life threatening, the misery they can cause by reducing a woman's self-esteem shouldn't be discounted. Intimate bonds with loving partners are fragile and easily broken in mid-life when other changes take place, so being unable to enjoy intercourse should not be tolerated.

Vaginal oestrogens effectively relieve common vulvovaginal symptoms and have additional effects on urinary symptoms such as urinary urgency, frequency or nocturia, stress urinary incontinence (SUI), and recurrent urinary tract infections (UTIs).

If you've already decided that you will not take HRT, or you cannot due to other health reasons, then you need to prepare for GSM. Moisturising the vulva regularly with non-hormonal moisturizers from your early 40s and stretching your vagina with a dildo (if you have no partner) will be good habits to adopt and continue.

The symptoms of genitourinary syndrome of menopause (GSM) include: -

- Vaginal dryness before/during sex
- Vaginal discomfort or pain during sex
- Vaginal itching and/or burning
- Itching or irritation on the outer lips or labia
- Frequent or re-occurring vaginal or urinary infections
- Thrush-like symptoms
- Lack of bladder control

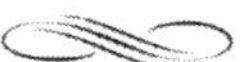

When intercourse is painful, you're naturally more likely to make excuses to your partner; but there is a danger that if you don't resolve this problem, your desire for sex and the consequent closeness to your partner is diminished. If you think that this problem is yours and yours alone, then of course, you might be too embarrassed to discuss it with your partner, especially if there is **smelly discharge**. Feeling guilty and frustrated is normal, so I urge you to understand that this symptom is common and is easily resolved. If you don't want to discuss it with your male doctor then book an appointment with the nurse or even a healthcare assistant – any of them will be able to talk things through and if you want them to, arrange a prescription for you.

This is actually one of the simplest problems to fix, and your doctor can get you a natural (soy or yam extract) containing an extremely low-dose oestrogen supplement in the form of a gel, a vaginal pessary or a soft doughnut-like ring. The gel is used externally on the vulva, other options are used internally. This works for the majority of women who try it by improving the quality of skin within the vagina, making it better lubricated and thicker.

Even if you suffer from bleeding classed as heavy for long periods, you can still use the vaginal ring which delivers a steady dose of oestrogen for up to 12 weeks.

I have a friend who uses the vaginal pessaries and, after initial treatment of using it every day for two weeks, she now only inserts it twice a week. She had suffered several infections which felt a lot like cystitis, but anti-biotics or anti-fungal type treatment didn't clear them up. Her doctor eventually prescribed *Vagifem* pessaries and my friend is so happy, feels confident and clean again; more than that, intercourse is back on the menu. There is no evidence that this type of oestrogen supplement raises the level of oestrogen systemically and has low potential to encourage any development of cancer or blood clots. If you already have hormone therapy and still have vaginal symptoms, this can be **added into your plan** to prevent you needing to increase the dose of hormones you already use.

If you truly don't want any added oestrogen to your body, there are other options.

If you have had breast cancer and have persistent troublesome genital or vaginal symptoms which aren't improving with vaginal moisturizers and lubricants, local oestrogen treatment may be a possibility. Your Urogynecologist can co-ordinate the use of vaginal oestrogen with your Oncologist. Studies so far have not shown an increased risk of cancer recurrence in women using vaginal oestrogen who are undergoing treatment of breast cancer or those with history of breast cancer. Of course, if you're unfortunate to have had double mastectomy, this type of supplement will cause no harm.

Lubricants are also helpful and not just before intercourse; used regularly you'll feel more comfortable. Water based non-perfumed products are best and the brands called Sylk, Yes and Replens have a good selection. Make sure the one you use is organic, paraben-free, glycerine-free and pH-balanced. You can use these daily as moisturisers, applied regularly, they can be very helpful and may stave off worse problems later on.

We moisturise our faces, hands and bodies, but when we miss a few days, they still feel dry, and the skin always thins with age. All through our lives we moisturise. Except our vulva and vaginas, which we expect to remain soft, strong and flexible through tampon use, sex, and childbirth. So, show a little love for your genitals and start moisturising every day. Just as a side note, chemotherapy treatment can also be the cause of vaginal problems.

Dildos can be used (where there is no alternative) to keep your vaginal passage lubricated and the tissues around the cervix healthy. In the absence of a partner, you can find any size of product at many different price points via internet sites.

A friend of mine told me that she met a new partner at the age of 62, after several years of no intercourse. When they had sex for the first time, she was shocked to feel pain as though his penis was ripping her open. She did some research and bought a small dildo and some lubricant and re-trained her vagina to accept a penis, then she bought a bigger dildo!

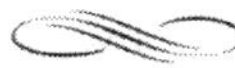

VAGINAL NIP & TUCK

Emerging treatments using laser and radiofrequency energy are gaining popularity in patients who will pay privately for a tightening of their vagina and for patients who have experienced prolapse. These treatments are similar to the ablations used in the treatment of very heavy menstrual bleeding. They have been developed to enhance the look and structure of your vulva and vagina.

Procedures which are cosmetic in nature are not easily available via NHS or medical insurance, but if you have suffered a vaginal prolapse, you're a good patient for these treatments which tighten the vaginal walls.

Genital rejuvenation may become the next frontier in medical and cosmetic dermatology, offering rejuvenation of the vagina and scrotum. Rejuvenation of the genitalia may be considered for hair-associated (alopecia and hypertrichosis), morphology-associated (vulvovaginal atrophy, excess clitoral or labial tissue, scrotal wrinkling, and vaginal or scrotal laxity), and vascular-associated (angiokeratomas) changes of the vagina and scrotum.

Radiofrequency Devices emit focused electromagnetic waves that heat underlying tissues. Within the vagina, they produce thermal energy which encourages new collagen fibre production, the tightening of existing collagen fibres, and the production of new blood vessels into areas which may have lost blood flow. All of which helps in restoring the elasticity and moisture of the vaginal lining.

Laser devices can do the same as radiofrequency devices. If you've ever investigated facial treatments which use lasers, then you'll have some understanding of what happens.

There is little evidence from clinical trials that this type of treatment works, outside of an operating theatre. Several clinics have popped up to offer treatments, but the reviews from clients are mainly that the treatment has only a moderate effect and needs regular topping up sessions. The cost per session is around £400 and a course of three is recommended to begin with.

Outside of the operating theatre, these clinics are regulated by the Care Quality Council insofar as to ensure the machines are used and stored safely; the CQC offer no approval to the actual procedures.

The above are both internal treatments and involve a probe being inserted to your vagina and the magic happens. Both can improve the frictional forces which increase sexual sensation. Private clinics suggest that stress incontinence can be relieved using laser therapy, but all women are different, and the results are variable.

Stem cell therapy is a treatment which involves removing adipose tissue (also known as fat) from your body and extracting stem cells from within that tissue. These stem cells are treated and prepared to be reintroduced to your body as adipose tissue rich with adipose stem cells. The fact that these cells are your own means they will be accepted within the cell structure of your vulva and vagina, and will go to work on improving the look, texture, and contours within those areas.

This procedure is called lipofilling and is an efficient treatment to restore soft tissue volume. It is mainly used in aesthetic and reconstructive surgery. It can also be used on the face as a non-surgical face lift and reconstruction technique. Many years ago, when I worked as a clinical aromatherapist, I had a client who had some areas where the underlying tissue of her face had lost volume. I was unable to help her using aromatherapy, but this technique of lipofilling would possibly have worked for her.

Lipofilling is being used with great success, alongside corrective surgery, on young women who have suffered genital mutilation. I'm honoured to know Aurora Almadori, RCS, a leading surgeon in London Free Hospital, who is pioneering this work.

Other techniques include the use of growth factors from your own blood. This latter technique is called PRP (platelet-rich plasma).

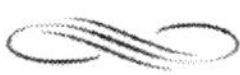

VULVAL LICHEN

Although this next issue isn't necessarily a symptom of menopause, it's a rarely discussed issue which a few women develop. I thought that while we're on the subject of vaginas, we should discuss it here.

Vulval lichen sclerosus (LS) and Vulval lichen planus (LP) are conditions that affect the skin of the vulva. For a very few women LS or LP can develop into a type of skin cancer called squamous cell cancer, which can take many years to develop.

Symptoms of LS or LP can include itchy, sore or fragile skin around the vulva, which may have changed in colour. Because very few women actually examine themselves in this area, it may go undetected unless there is discomfort in the outer vaginal lips when having sex or passing urine. If you notice any of these signs, go and see your GP who will examine you and probably refer you to a specialist for further tests.

Lipofilling has an added benefit for the woman who suffers Vulval lichen sclerosus (LS) or Vulval lichen planus (LP). The regenerative effect of stem cell therapy has been shown to heal the scars caused by this problematic symptom.

Until recently the perception was that LS and LP can be treated but can't be completely cured. As we discover from the above trial with stem cell therapy, this could have changed. The usual treatment will be a steroid ointment which can often control the symptoms very well.

Neither of these symptoms are infectious and cannot be passed on through sex. If you think you may have a problem and intend to make an appointment to see your GP, ask for a nurse or other female to be with you during examination. Tell your doctor if you develop any symptoms you are concerned about, such as a lump or swelling, or any itching, bleeding or burning pain.

The causes of LS and LP are unknown, although some women with these conditions have other family members with either, so perhaps it may be caused by an inherited faulty gene. Both issues are more common in older women and women who have autoimmune illnesses, such as thyroid problems or pernicious anaemia.

Women who've had LS or LP for many years have a small risk of developing a vulval cancer. This usually occurs in women in their 60s–90s, rather than in younger women. It's important to see your doctor or nurse regularly to check for any signs of a cancer developing. This is so that if cancer does develop, treatment can be given at an early stage, when there's a high chance of it being cured.

SEX IN MENOPAUSE

I'm not going to lie to you here, I still enjoy sex and intimacy. Like most children, I could hear what my parents were doing through the bedroom walls and have to admit it scared me a bit. As a teenager, I absolutely flat out didn't want to consider my parents still having sex, even though I could still hear the activity!

As for myself, a different story that might be told later, but I grew up feeling unsafe around men and absolutely terrified of putting myself in a situation where the person I was with expected intercourse. (So much so that a dear friend nicknamed me 'frigid Fred' which hurt me very much when I found out). This had nothing to do with the embarrassment of my tiny underdeveloped breasts and everything to do with vulnerability.

Now I'm at this beautiful age, having a fulfilling intimate relationship is as good as breathing deeply, it's relaxing and satisfying. It makes my eyes glow and I'm more relaxed, physically. So what if my body isn't what it was and my wrinkles hang proudly when I'm on top, my partner has aged as well, so we're even.

And, I have to say that solo sex is every bit as good, different, but good. In a tired or busy life, pleasing yourself is lovely, quick and very satisfying.

Intimacy isn't always about sex, and having sex is not necessarily intimate. Huh? Let's use the word intercourse instead of sex because that word defines what most of us think of when we discuss sex. When you had your first full relationship where intercourse happened regularly, did you think that gentle touching and tender voices were sexy or intimate? Did you think it was important to be intimate, or was being sexy all that mattered?

The difference is subtle but important and I'll tell you why. I have a dear friend who has been married over 40 years and she told me recently that she still loves her husband "and can't get enough of him". When I'm with her and her partner, I feel loved as well, because they are so generous with their loving that everyone else shares it. I've been in the company of other couples who can excite each other with just a look, a smile or a gentle touch; this is intimacy. It's the shared joke, shared history, shared plans and dreams. It's feeling total trust that your partner will never hurt you, (especially with words) so that you become more and more open to your real authentic self, which helps the trust between you to grow even greater. You can feel beloved just because your partner strokes your shoulder as they walk past.

However, when you lack personal confidence it's easy to slip out of sexy and into self-judgement. You can become anxious about your rolls of fat or facial wrinkles or skin texture on your bum and thighs, or whatever is your personal hang-up. Judging yourself this way is sure to kill the vibe of intimacy. Once you believe that you're not good enough, you'll subconsciously pass that belief onto your partner and open the door for a level of behaviour from them that is less than you should accept. Not every partner will take advantage of that, but it's human/animal nature that whenever anyone puts themselves into a position of subservience, the other will rise higher.

In the seventies I had my own beauty salon and my favourite treatment was massage because I loved knowing that touch is healing. I had male clients who were, in the main, respectful. However, I knew that if any thoughts of desire or anything sensual entered my head, then he would pick up on that, and the vibe would change instantly; I know this because very occasionally it happened. We all know that having a loving and fulfilling sexual relationship is optimum in a long-term relationship, but what happens when that isn't what you get, or when your relationship changes and intimacy go out of the door.

For many women around peri menopause onwards, this part of loving can be the last item on the list of things to do. Planning to have children in her thirties means having teenagers who need extra emotional support just when Mum is living through her own hormonal tornado. Add into this a career that needs to continue for financial reasons, or because she loves her work, elderly parents who need some support, oh and finally, a partner who doesn't really understand where his woman disappeared to.

Doctors who specialise in female health will say that it's very common for women to have problems with their libido around menopause. Those women will regularly feel guilty about this, especially if they have previously enjoyed a good sexual relationship. It isn't many generations ago that women would not expect to be still sexually active in their 50s and 60s. Now that many women are living another third of their lives post menopause, we need to consider this as something to work on.

Sometimes all I need to feel loved is a beautiful hug, but for a man that can often be foreplay to sex, which I find exasperating, so I teach them. Recently I've found a global community who I connect with two or three times a year as a volunteer and we are all ages, shapes and orientation. One of the things I humbly regard as a service to other women is showing the younger men how to hug a woman so that she feels safe and loved and supported. If it's done well, this type of hug will build a level of intimacy so that intercourse may be welcome – later – not immediately after the hug.

Apart from situational reasons why you no longer have sex within your relationship, experiencing pain from intercourse is certain to make you not want it. If you do feel pain, you should gallop off to your doctor to check the symptoms. Please go to the chapter on Menopause Vagina to understand symptoms and remedies and take action.

Conversely, there are some women who report feeling they can't get enough sex and complain their partner can't keep up with them. Hormones eh? No rhyme or reason.

I am really struggling with my sex life! I have no libido. It's like something changed overnight! I have always been very, very horny, sorry for my crudeness. Spoke to my doc and she was no help at all. I am the other side of menopause for the past few years. 62 years old, I went through mild menopause. The usual night sweats, feeling low, lack of a good night sleep. Can't remember the last time I actually slept thru the night. Dry vagina just happened out of nowhere along with a wobbly tummy and love handles. My hubby is a few years older and is slowing down in the amazing erection days, but probably wouldn't mind a bit of the old enthusiasm from me. It's just not there! I miss the old days...

THYROID PROBLEMS

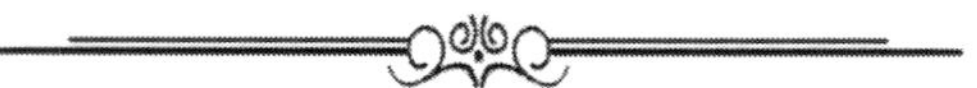

THE thyroid gland produces hormones and when it 'misbehaves' and puts those hormones out of balance, some of the symptoms produced are very similar to some of the symptoms of menopause. It is pretty common for thyroid gland problems to be discovered in women around the age of 40-50 which is when we are beginning the menopause. It seems that many women are living with undiagnosed thyroid problems, and it's only when we finally visit a health care professional to discuss menopause symptoms that a diagnosis is made.

One in eight women will develop thyroid problems in her lifetime.

My own story goes like this. I was 37 with a two-year-old son, the family farm was about to be sold and my husband would be without an income. At that point I'd been teaching aerobic exercise for several years and my classes were busy and popular.

In anticipation of the farm sale I opened a children's nursery which I hoped would generate enough income to support us while husband found his feet outside of farming. I then opened a second children's nursery and was feeling powerfully stressed because I was trying to do everything on a shoestring, and we know that being underfunded is not good for any new business. My family had membership of a lovely spa attached to a local hotel and we spent many hours there, my son learnt to swim in the pool and husband played in their squash league.

I'd begun to notice that I was very tired while swimming with my son and had started to just carry him on my back while I held onto the 'lip' of the pool and hauled myself around the perimeter.

During that summer we had house guests and we took them to the spa where husband and son went into the hot tub, and my friend and I swam a few lengths. However, I barely had the energy to reach the end and was breathless as I finally grabbed hold of the pool edge. That incident really frightened me, and I paid a visit to my GP who suggested that I take better care of my diet and try to rest more often.

That September I was invited to organise a new aerobics class in a different town, but during the first session my legs simply wouldn't work, my thigh muscles wouldn't lift my legs when we were jogging, and I was breathless after little effort. I returned to the GP who still didn't think anything was worth testing.

Other mysterious symptoms were surfacing:

- I had difficulty remembering what I was talking about and often was unable to finish a sentence or remember names, facts or details. Dealing with my clients at the nursery was pretty embarrassing because I didn't remember the names of their children who were in my care, let alone the names of the parents.
- I was deeply tired but couldn't sleep, I snored so much my husband sent me to the sofa.
- I was cold all the time, strangely the heel of my left hand felt as though it had an icicle within it.
- Emotionally I was a mess, completely out of control, tears and confusion.
- My hair had become dull and lifeless, coarse and thick, so I let it grow.
- My skin was thicker, and my complexion looked like cooked porridge, I could 'peel' my knuckles.
- Strangest to me was that my voice became deep and gruff which was drastic since all my life people had complimented me on my voice, even describing it as mellifluous.
- A relative suggested that my eyes were 'strange', slightly bulging and unfocussed.

- I had no appetite but when I did eat my body simply closed down and I had to sleep, noticeably I had some energy until I ate food, and then I collapsed.
- During this time my weight was fairly stable, although I noticed my waist was thicker, so I bought elastic waisted skirt and trousers.

At the end of one particular day, I closed up the nursery and headed for my evening aerobics class where I greeted my 30 or so clients, began the class but simply couldn't go on. I stopped the music, looked at them all, apologised and told them something was wrong, and while I didn't know what it was, I absolutely couldn't carry on and there'd be no more classes for a while.

That was the catalyst that caused my symptoms to overcome me, since I was no longer exercising, my body wasn't moving the lymph glands which keep the body clean of toxins, and every cell in my body began to stagnate.

My physical and emotional collapse was rapid, but I still had to care for my son and run the nursery, even though I had staff, the responsibility was only mine.

On a glorious blue-sky Sunday morning I was invited to go horse riding with a friend which was a lovely treat. We hacked up the hills above Ullswater and galloped the length of the old racetrack on top of Askham Fell; it was a memorable ride. I'd arranged to meet husband in the bar of the Spa where we had a chat and a half pint of lager.

We each had our own vehicles so agreed to meet at home for lunch and I drove away with him following close behind. I remember driving to the rear of our home and bringing my car to a halt but then nothing. I was woken by a knocking on the driver side window and opened my eyes to see a neighbour with a very worried expression on her face. She had come to find me to say that husband's car had been hit by a tractor and he was being taken to hospital. I hadn't even noticed that he wasn't behind me as I drove home.

This ability to stop driving and immediately fall into a deep sleep is still something I have to do, thirty years later. Before retirement I was working as a sales rep driving for hours at a time, I could be only ten minutes from home but had to stop for a nap.

Some months after I had ended my aerobics classes I was a wreck, barely able to stay awake but still trying to run my nursery business. The farm had been sold and husband, son and I had been removed to a farm cottage until we found somewhere of our choosing to live.

A chance meeting with an old **friend** was the trigger for me to go back to the GP. She stopped me in the street and told me how dreadful I looked, and she hoped I didn't mind, but she thought I could do with some help. Thank You. Finally, my GP took blood and after assuring me that my problem wasn't hormonal, he said that he would get me the results in a few days.

Two days later I was closing up the nursery and husband phoned to say that my GP needed to see me urgently and would wait for me. The surgery was a 45-minute drive away and it was already early evening, but apparently it was urgent. I locked the nursery and drove away.

I woke up on **a** lounger beside the pool at the spa, an attendant shook me awake and said my husband wanted to speak to me. I hurried to the telephone and husband very angrily asked me what I was doing? I'd totally blanked out after leaving the nursery and driven directly to the Spa, found a bed and fallen asleep.

This is what hormones can do to our systems when they go out of balance.

My discussion with the doctor next day went along the lines of "congratulations, you have one of the few health problems which will give you free prescriptions for life in the UK, take one of these pills every day and we'll see you in two months to see how you're doing". Shocking. The reason why the GP wanted to see me urgently and the reason why I was to have free prescriptions for life is that without thyroxine our bodies will die, simple; and I was slowly but surely dying.

The pills were thyroxine which is identical to what my own thyroid gland should have been producing, and within two months I looked, felt and spoke like my old self. Gradually I lost the extra weight I'd gained, and my energy returned. I cut my hair and really started to feel like me again, but I had been in very poor shape for almost a year before diagnosis and medication, and I still have little memory of those months.

WHY DOES A THYROID GLAND MISBEHAVE?

The most common cause of the thyroid gland going out of balance is because the body decides to attack it via the autoimmune system. The winter before diagnosis, husband and I simultaneously had really bad colds; or at least, I had a really heavy cold my husband had influenza! With no-one to help and a baby to care for I begged my GP for antibiotics and was given a course. I failed to finish that course of antibiotics and it's possible that was the cause of my immune system attacking my thyroid. That attack caused a reduction in my production of thyroid stimulating hormone, or TSH, which should have told my pituitary gland to continue production of a balanced amount of thyroxine.

For more information on thyroid problems and helpful support, go to: http://www.thyroiduk.org.uk

TROPICAL MOMENTS & NIGHTSWEATS

I'm still hot

THE MOST DREADED of all the menopausal symptoms, the hot flushes (or flashes) and night sweats. This is the symptom which can cause huge misery and despair amongst women and yet, some women barely notice them.

The first few times this happens, you might feel anxious if your heart begins to beat faster, then you feel heat creeping all over your body until your scalp and top lip feel sweaty. These could begin in your early 40s and if you don't expect it, you might worry that you're having a panic attack or worse, a heart attack. Some women don't experience them through the day but wake in the night wet from sweating and occasionally wet from urine. It feels a bit like when you have a heavy cold and are feverish, that's the general feeling.

Why does this happen? It's our friend oestrogen making a slow but sure retreat from the gland in the brain called the hypothalamus which regulates body temperature. When the hypothalamus goes out of balance it can get the wrong signal telling it your body is overheating. In order to bring your body temperature back to normal, this gland tells the whole body to sweat to get rid of the heat, that's when you develop a hot flush or night sweat. Horrid, yes. Fixable, possibly.

It seems to be a symptom that is 'western' in that the Japanese don't recognise hot flushes as relevant within menopause, they don't even have a name for the symptom in Japanese. This is possibly because the 'Eastern' woman has eaten soy regularly over her whole lifetime, but some women I've spoken to in the West have found that eating soy or drinking soymilk helps to reduce the number of times this happens each day.

There are other lifestyle choices which seem to trigger extra hot flushes for some women. Those are eating spicy foods, drinking fizzy soft drinks or alcohol; especially drinking anything with caffeine in. That includes any cold medicine containing caffeine. For a better night's sleep and fewer hot flushes through the day, cut out caffeine completely, if you can. Smoking is also a trigger.

Exercise will help but, if you don't get enough sleep because of the night sweats, you're unlikely to feel like doing any; however, it gives your body something else to think about. The positive emotional satisfaction when you've finished a run or yoga session or whatever, can be really supportive.

My own hot flushes were especially troublesome when I had to speak in public, either in a team meeting or in front of the company, sometimes just with one client. I would feel warm around the head and knew that I had the blotchy mess around my neck and chest, not very attractive. I didn't realise this was related to menopause until much later when it stopped happening, I just thought I was anxious about public speaking.

Here are a few comments from other women struggling with 'tropical moments'

> *'Want to ask if my hot flushes are normal or if anyone else is like this. my heart starts to flutter I get so hot it lasts for 20mins, get breathless like anxiety attack so I put fan on. once it's past I'm cold? I have them about 6 times a day. I'm having more anxiety attacks when I go shopping and flush so much.'*

'This seems very back to front. Was having hot flushes a hell of a lot but since my last period 2 months ago they seem to have gone. But this week I've been so cold, I just can't get warm. Do any of you think that maybe you're not actually going through the menopause, I feel like everything is in my head at times.'

'My second night of no hot flushes. It may be a fluke but I'm keeping my fingers crossed. I can't take HRT so have to rely on homeopathic remedies. I take menopause original that doesn't work, but I'm frightened to come off in case my symptoms get worse. but after watching the informative programme that the BBC did on menopause, I've started drinking Soya milk. I drink just under a litre a day and it truly is helping. I'm more myself than I've been in years, I still have the odd bad day, but I really do feel it's helping, maybe it would help other girls who are suffering too.'

'I'm getting a definite increase in hot flushes, I'm 40 days in with the sertraline and wondering if there could be a connection, or coincidence? Meanwhile the sertraline is doing its job and I've lost the general fear, dread and sense of horror that was so normal, I hadn't realised how much it was there. I'm having different dreams, all healing the past stuff. All good.'

'I'm 55 and I guess going through the Menopause. I haven't had hot flushes; I get night sweats. My GP point blank refused HRT but gave me Vagifem around 5 years ago which I still take twice a week. Have any of you been prescribed this... The Nurse Practitioner told me that it's better than HRT?'

'Ultimately it's your choice but your GP is letting herself down by not giving you up to date facts. I am generally appalled at GPs quoted on here, including one of mine. I have found male medical staff much more empathetic. Especially a mature male GP who clearly has personal experience of treating and living with menopause. Personally, I have gone through hell with truly debilitating symptoms. A week today I will be heading home post hysterectomy with HRT patches in my bag and getting my life back. I will not be coming off them anytime soon'

Many women would truly be grateful for an arrangement where they can sleep alone during this time of their life; not to say they don't want to snuggle up to their partner for a kiss goodnight or good morning.

It's just that playing hokey-cokey with arms and legs can be a problem. That and being so wet around the chest and between the legs, is not so lovely. If you can't have a run-away bedroom, then perhaps the biggest bed you can fit into the room is another option. Using low thread-count pure cotton or linen sheets, separate duvets, a cool gel pad beneath your side of the mattress, a cold-water bottle, wearing light cotton pjs and a cool bedroom are all good suggestions.

There is a ton of suggestions for the relief of night sweats and hot flushes, supplementing your oestrogen with an appropriate dose is the most successful, but if you cannot or don't want to do that then I have more options within the 'Treatments & Remedies' chapter.

WEIGHT

loving what is

WHEN I OWNED my beauty therapy salon in the 1970s, I specialised in body treatments for slimming purposes. I could tell if a client had lost or gained weight just by looking at her, and I still notice if a woman (who I know) has gained or lost weight just by looking at her.

Therefore, I can tell you that there's a kind of 'over blown' or 'blowsiness' to women who are entering the early months of menopause. That often involves weight gain around the middle, from the breasts down, and just like mine, it seems to happen overnight. One day I had a fairly flat tummy and almost the next day I looked as though I'd eaten pasta daily for a month.

I can remember when this happened to me and I asked my healthcare nurse why? she shrugged and gave me the usual response of 'it's just your age'. I laughed and asked her 'why, when my body is no longer able to create and carry a baby, do I now need fat around my abdomen which looks as though it's protecting my reproductive organs?' She just laughed. Of course, I now know why this happens, and I'm going to tell you in a minute. Uncommon is weight gain around the thighs or arms, even though both those areas may look bigger due to loss of muscle tone. Experts agree that as we age into our forties, our bodies are not so good at using the food we eat as energy and we store what we don't use as fat, we all know this.

Now because of this, over an average year without any change in our diet, we add on around one pound in weight per year. Which means that over the ten years of peri and menopause (say between 47 and 57) we might gain around ten pounds by doing absolutely nothing different. Fair? I don't think so, and the worse news is that the body is less willing to let go of that weight, so we have to exercise harder just to maintain our usual weight. Ten pounds is a dress size, if you like. I can remember going to a friend's fiftieth birthday party and being asked afterwards if I'd had my breasts enlarged. Funny? not really, but at the time, being able to totally fill a bra was the only thing I was grateful to my menopause for.

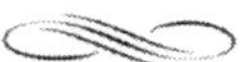

How much extra risk do we put ourselves in by gaining weight before and through menopause, and not losing it afterwards? Great question, because we know that excess weight increases the risk of heart disease, type 2 diabetes, breathing problems and various types of cancer, including colon, endometrial and especially breast cancer.

Diabetes is classified into two types. A person with type 1 diabetes will usually be diagnosed in childhood or teenage years; they are always dependant on daily injections of insulin. A person with type 2 diabetes is normally diagnosed in later life, and the cause of it is usually either life choices or old age. If a person is unable to control their type 2 diabetes through changing their life choices, they will be given medication to support their body's ability to use insulin. Doctors know that each 5 unit increase in body mass index (BMI) is linked to a 60-100% increased risk of developing bladder incontinence.

The World Health Organisation has decreed that a woman with a waist measurement of 35 inches or more is obese, in any language. *Being overweight or obese is the greatest risk to developing breast cancer in middle life and is actually 6x the risk to this type of cancer than taking hormone therapy.*

This is because fat cells also make their own oestrogen, and therefore an obese woman will continue to make oestrogen after her ovaries stop making it. All studies show that the longer a woman has oestrogen in her body, the higher the risk of developing breast cancer.

Other factors, such as a lack of exercise, unhealthy eating, and not enough sleep, might contribute to menopause weight gain. When we don't get enough sleep, we tend to unconsciously snack more and consume more calories. If we include the loss of self-esteem caused by hot flushes, memory loss and bladder weakness, it's hardly a surprise that many women feel constantly under threat and enjoy a glass or two of wine after work. Cortisol is released by the brain when we're stressed and having cortisol in the blood stream is associated with increased appetite, cravings for sugar and of course, weight gain.

I've mentioned previously about my own years of depression, and one thing I've noticed is the effect that being under stress has on my weight. I know that if I'm 'happy stressed' because I'm excited, for example have fallen in love, (heady days) then I lose a few pounds. However, in a work scenario when I'm being poorly managed, or a relationship isn't going well, then I can become 'worried stressed' and that has caused me to add on several pounds very quickly. Now I understand about the effect cortisol has on weight balance, I completely understand why.

In other conversations women told me they were afraid of taking hormone therapy because they didn't want to gain weight, but just as many women lose weight when they take hormone therapy as gain it. Being blunt, I think it's inevitable that you will add on some weight with or without supplementing your natural oestrogen, whichever way you choose to supplement it. Even our 'National Treasure' the very beautiful Twiggy has changed shape during her menopause.

Listen, what I suggest is that you STOP beating yourself up about growing older and experiencing body changes, you will change. Never, ever forget that any man who is lucky enough to have his arms around you in or out of bed WILL NEVER EVER COMPLAIN if you are a smidgeon chunkier than when he met you. If he's a new friend then he was attracted to YOU, full stop. I doubt that he'll complain when you get down to skin, but If he does and he's not joking, feel free to remove yourself from his embrace but not before you give his 'beer belly' or his bald head, or his flabby backside, a prod with a very strong finger.

Women going through menopause are very often struggling with other major life changes such as children leaving home or returning, divorce, death of loved ones and trying to plan their retirement. While I'm not offering excuses for anyone who gains weight, I am suggesting that women as a group should treat themselves with a lot more love.

Why do we add on weight especially around the middle? The answer is (possibly) that we produce around twice as much testosterone during our lives than we produce oestrogen (surprise!). However, when we go through menopause the production of testosterone gradually decreases, whereas the production of oestrogen slows down and eventually stops fairly abruptly, leaving an imbalance in favour of testosterone. This is why the fat we gain is stored in a more typically male (beer belly) style and I personally began to look as though I drank three pints of beer every night. Supplementing your hormones correctly will re-distribute that fat and help to relieve the problem of central or 'visceral' weight gain, which will help with many of the health issues mentioned above.

Most of the women I spoke to felt that they would be unable to lose the extra weight gained during menopause because 'everyone knows that's impossible'. Over the years since my own menopause I also had decided that it was impossible because I'd 'tried' and 'failed' and still had my beer belly. However, I'm ecstatic to tell you that it is actually possible to lose that weight in a healthy and meaningful way which will not just reappear next month.

My belief, however, is that you won't be totally successful until your hormones are settled. I don't have any scientific proof of this, but I am living proof and know several women who also succeeded. Saying that, it shouldn't be an excuse to not keep your weight relatively balanced because the benefits of being lighter are huge.

Moderate helpings are good because, (experts say) we all eat too much at a time. Apparently, the volume of each meal should be no bigger than the volume of your fist, and that makes some sense because your stomach (although very elastic) is actually quite small. Make green foods your friend and fill up on them rather than beige foods such as potatoes, pasta and bread. Snack foods don't need to be in your larder all the time either, like crisps, salted nuts, popcorn or processed (full of additives, but tasty) meat products.

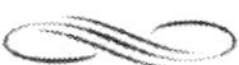

Two things happened which made me take a very different approach to having a healthier weight. The first was that I visited a 78-year-old friend who had been warned by her clinician that she was at risk of developing type 2 diabetes and had fairly quickly dropped fourteen pounds to ensure she stayed healthy.

The second was that I went to a personal development event during which we did an exercise to create our own 'wheel of life'. This exercise is designed to highlight areas of life where I was or was not satisfied, i.e. love or career or financial. When I looked at the wheel I had created, my first thought was that my physical body was something I could take control of and improve almost immediately. With the example of my friend in mind and the certain knowledge that my fatty spare tyre was doing dreadful things to my vital organs, I shocked my body into giving up all that fat.

I make no claim towards being a nutritionist and this is not advice, but I'm just going to tell you what I did. Two years before this weight loss I had a deeply unpleasant disagreement with some wild mushrooms and the consequence of that was I stopped eating meat (I know it makes no sense, but my taste changed). I still eat fish and meat substitutes but no chicken or red meat.

I had changed my diet a few times previously with little affect, but this time I decided to shock my body with a totally different way of eating. This is sometimes described as 'biohacking'** your body. Twenty years earlier I was living through a deeply painful divorce, and the physical affect was that my digestive system was out of control. I had gas, my stools were either very loose or I was constipated; generally, it was a result of stress. I resolved the problem by 'biohacking'** my system - removing white carbohydrates and root vegetables from my diet, just to see what would happen. Twenty years ago, this approach worked and my digestion re-set itself. In my sixties I wondered if this approach would work again.

By the way, this isn't any particular diet or way of eating, it's just what I hoped might work for me. I tripled the amount of green vegetables I ate and continued to enjoy my morning porridge with fresh fruit and honey. Substituting some of my dairy with coconut 'milk' in my porridge was also an ok choice. There are so many alternatives available that we never need to feel deprived of dairy.

I made smoothies with yoghurt made from coconut, fruit and honey; and green smoothies with apple juice, spinach, kale, fresh ginger, fennel, mint and avocado (whatever was available). To add protein, I put maccha powder in to all my smoothies, which is also widely available. I found a terrific vitamin and mineral supplement which has given me huge amounts of energy and great mental health. I wasn't avoiding fat, just eating quality fat (oil from avocado, coconut and flax, plus butter and cheese from grass fed cows) instead of synthetics like low-fat spread and no fat yoghurt.

By removing yeast and sugar from my diet, my digestion immediately improved, and the bloated feeling followed soon after. Two years later my weight loss has balanced itself out and my face has filled back out again. During that change in my eating pattern, I noticed that I rarely felt hungry, and I think that has something to do with not telling myself I was on a diet. I told myself that I was making healthier choices, that I was making a deliberate and considered decision about not eating certain foods. It was a *preference* to lose weight and be fitter, rather than *pressure*.

Some women are reluctant to lose weight just because they might start to look facially 'haggard' but for me I didn't care. I reasoned that if men weren't interested in me when my face was beautifully plump, then what would change if it wasn't. Plus, I felt so much better it was a revelation. I now spend some of my day feeling hungry, and it's really good. I have a lightness to my body and my thoughts, and as much energy as a thirty-year-old.

Now that my hormones have re-adjusted and my weight seems stable, I've added back into my diet some root vegetables, occasional cake, and cheese. What I do notice these days is that when I eat sugar, either in wine or desserts or cakes, I immediately see the effect in fluid retention, which makes me a little 'puffy' around my middle. So that's something I'm aware of.

When I want to be sure I can get into a bikini or my favourite denim, I pay attention to what I'm eating (or am mindful of what I eat) and stay away from empty sugar calories. Although there's a school of thought that any sugar in a glass of wine could be regarded as menopause medicine.

As well as weight loss, many women notice that a change in their diet brings some relief from symptoms of menopause, particularly hot flushes and night sweats. I've read lots of reports that avoiding spicy food, cutting right back on alcohol and caffeine, and stopping smoking all help with this. I'm sure you'll agree that getting a few hours quality sleep goes a long way to make up for the loss of a nightcap whether it's coffee or alcohol. Those women also reported that reducing or removing sugar from their diet helped in reducing hot flushes and night sweats as well, it reduces food cravings of all kinds – I don't know why it does, but it does.

biohacking is a relatively new word for "changing your environment from the inside out so that you have full control over your biology, using your body as your personal laboratory to find the exact hacks that work for you". It was created by Dave Asprey who, following a severe brain injury, discovered that drinking coffee with butter worked some magic on his brain and led to him writing a book called* ***Head Strong*. That book was followed by others and he's now a thought leader in nutrition. I would recommend reading his books simply to challenge your beliefs about 'diet'. Biohacking should be a temporary diet and not to be considered as the way you'll eat for the rest of your life. Having said that, if your new approach to nutrition is successful for you, why would you choose to go back to eating the things that made you feel bloated or sluggish or mentally dull?*

PART TWO

TELL ME ALL ABOUT IT

Never be afraid or embarrassed to discuss symptoms

It's very common for women to miss the first signs of menopause because they just aren't expecting it. We're educated to believe that we will be in menopause in our early 50s, but no one I've spoken to has been educated to understand that perimenopause (marking the slowing down of oestrogen production) starts in our early 40s. The first sign that your body is changing might be that you begin to have night sweats, or your periods change and become heavier or less regular.

You may visit the clinic because even though you've never had premenstrual tension symptoms before, they develop in your mid-40s. Or, if you do have regular PMS it becomes much worse and feels just like the irritability and irrationality of a teenager. You may become angry, paranoid, deeply anxious have panic attacks, or develop migraine attacks for the first time in your forties, as I did.

There may be constant and dreadful tiredness, which feels as though your body simply closes down and your 'life force' drains away.

Regularly needing to rest during the day is partly caused by sleep deprivation due to night sweats. You may develop aching joints that feels like flu, or find you have terrible concentration levels and poor memory for names and nouns.

Many women manage their physical symptoms well but when they lose libido, drive and motivation, have no will to live, can no longer multitask, and lose their ability to cope well with complex lives, then they look for the support of their doctor.

For some, a visit to their doctor is simply to confirm what they're thinking; that they are going through the menopause and not actually having a breakdown or developing some kind of disorder. Often, they simply want a conversation around the issues and to understand why they feel so different.

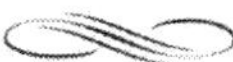

A recent report from the British Menopause Society informs us that women believe they will experience, on average, seven symptoms of the menopause which will last around four years. Also, they feel that because this is just a part of life every woman goes through, then they have to put up with those symptoms.

The reality is that for most women, the early symptoms of perimenopause such as difficulty sleeping, chaotic menstruation, hot flushes, mood swings and joint ache will last between five and seven years. But for one in ten women, some of those debilitating symptoms can last up to twelve years.

It's my opinion that those years between forty-five and sixty can and should be the most glorious years for a woman, and twelve years of symptoms is too much to just put up with when it means a significant reduction in the quality of life during those years.

However, a new survey has revealed that nearly half of women going through the menopause suffer in silence and avoid discussing their symptoms with the doctor because they are too embarrassed.

Unfortunately, and I can only speak about medical care in the UK, it is rare to find a health clinic or surgery where a member of the team specialises in or has an interest in menopause. During the writing of this book I spoke to many women at various stages of their menopause. Many of them were underwhelmed, or even distressed by the response from their doctor.

Sadly, some doctors will listen to the list of symptoms and placate the patient with a 'well, it's that time of life', or 'you're sad because the children are leaving home', or, 'you're not coping with your elderly parent', and even 'I think you have a level of depression' (they look at a scale of depression chart, tick, tick tick). This often results in women being given a prescription for anti-depressants to calm down or to aid sleep, and that can deepen her feeling of low self-worth or failure.

Anti-depressant treatment can work well in the reduction of some emotional symptoms, but it won't address the physical symptoms caused by lack of oestrogen. This misdiagnosis is why I've written this book, to empower you to take charge of your own health and to be informed about your menopause.

It seems that the majority of women don't understand their options around the menopause and, when the symptoms show up, they can feel powerless because of the generations of mythology and fear that surrounds treatment.

What is the menopause and how do you know that you're over it/starting it/going through it?

To make this part simple, I'm going to break it up into age groups because the treatment you'll be offered, and the advice given will depend on your age. In the UK the average age of a woman IN her menopause is 51, and she will have been going through peri menopause for a few years before that.

Female hormones, what why and how is something that most women think about during their life. Usually the question is around who designed us and what joke were they playing when they decided to create us with so many hormones that increase and decrease as we age; leaving us 'out of balance' for more than half of our lives.

Here's what I know; the main hormones which manage a woman's fertility (and that's the only reason we have puberty and periods) are progesterone and oestrogens (also sometimes called estrogens). As our bodies start to manufacture these hormones, we go through puberty so that we can become pregnant. There is then a length of time (around 30 years) when they ebb and flow during which we either become pregnant or not.

As the number of eggs, we carry dwindles, those hormones begin to disappear from our bodies as their manufacture and release slows down. While the manufacturing process is in decline our bodies are going through the perimenopause, (around 6-10 years). You are still potentially able to become pregnant but at an age when it's not common unless 'accidental'. Once the fertility hormone factory closes altogether, you're in the menopause and no longer able to become pregnant spontaneously.

However, the group of hormones called oestrogens is responsible for the health of a large number of systems other than your reproductive one. Oestrogens also maintain the balanced function of our brain, muscles, skin, hair, digestion and around 200 more physical areas. This is why we can feel so 'not like ourselves', or 'out of balance' or just 'off' when oestrogen production slows down and disappears. Those systems we should be most concerned about keeping in great health are cardiovascular (heart), skeletal (bones), and digestion (to prevent type 2 diabetes).

It is rare, but some 20-year olds can enter perimenopause; there isn't a particular reason why they do but it happens. For a very young woman this must be bewildering. The symptoms are exactly as described for a 40-year-old so if you know a young woman who is struggling, please give her your support and share this book.

If you are aged 45 or less and have some of the symptoms described in this book, you may be given a blood test to measure your FSH or follicle stimulating hormone. This hormone is responsible for preparing the ovary to produce an egg and if the blood test shows that the level is high it means you have a low amount of oestrogen available. The negative side of this blood test is that if you are in perimenopause, your oestrogen production will be fluctuating daily, therefore, the blood test may not give an accurate reading. So, the nurse/doctor may ask you to take a second blood test around 4-6 weeks later to double check the first result.

The reason why this blood test is done for women below the age of 45 is because it can be used to measure premature ovarian insufficiency (POI). POI is not common, but can be misdiagnosed, so if you have some symptoms of perimenopause, do get yourself checked over.

Premature ovarian insufficiency is usually diagnosed by these symptoms: -

1. No or infrequent periods for more than 3 months
2. Raised FSH (follicle stimulating hormone)
3. Low oestradiol levels (oestradiol is the main one of 3 hormones in the group called oestrogens)
4. Age below 45

When POI is diagnosed it means that fertility is reduced, and women may find getting pregnant is not possible or takes far longer than usual. However, you should still use contraception unless you're trying to be pregnant. The UK guidelines are that you should continue to use contraception until age 51 which is the average natural age when menopause is complete.

As previously said, females need oestrogen to maintain the best health of our skin, muscles, bones, brain, hair, digestive system and much more, so it's no surprise that if a woman is diagnosed with POI the advice is that she should consider taking the combined contraceptive pill to support all of those systems for continued good health. OR if she decides to take an alternative route, she needs to be ultra-diligent with the very best diet and exercise regime for many years.

Drinking alcohol most days, being overweight, smoking and leading an inactive life will very likely put the body at higher risk of stroke, heart attack, osteoporosis and type 2 diabetes. Taking HRT in the form of the combined contraceptive pill from an early age is considered to be 'no risk' because you're just replacing the hormones that your body should be producing itself, and many women who start taking it in early forties report few menopausal symptoms. Switching to HRT post menopause, they stay healthy and fit through their fifties and sixties and prefer to stay on hormone therapy for as long as they can.

If you are aged over 45, are experiencing some of the symptoms listed in this book, and have had irregular periods for several months, you're probably in perimenopause, which is the transition into full menopause. In the UK you won't need a blood test to confirm it, but this may be different in other parts of the world.

You may not be in a relationship and have no chance of engaging in sex between now and next Christmas, but hormonal contraception is still the best bridge from perimenopause to menopause. You need to discuss your family health history and any concerns you have, think about questions before you go, and ask your Mother or Aunts about historic family illness you may not know about.

You will probably be offered some type of hormone therapy which is additional oestrogen and progesterone to protect your body's systems described above, as well as to relieve the symptoms you're experiencing. This depends on what hormonal contraception you already use, if any. If this suits you, then you can stay on this combined contraception therapy until through the menopause or you are no longer fertile. See below.

You need to understand what hormone therapy is, how it works and what are the benefits of taking it. I discuss all of this later in the chapter on Treatments/Remedies. Hormone therapy is the number one treatment of choice, in most developed countries, to manage menopausal symptoms and to maintain optimum long-term health. You should discuss any of your health history that might make this unsuitable for you with the clinician. For example, previous blood clot, deep vein thrombosis, high blood pressure, do you smoke, are you overweight, family history of any of the above or breast cancer.

If you haven't had a period for 12 months and you are aged 51 or older when you first visit your clinic then it's assumed that you're through perimenopause and actually into menopause. The need for contraception is over because it's rare that a woman will spontaneously become fertile at this age. However, talking through your choices of oestrogen and progesterone hormone replacement with your clinician is important for long term health and protection.

Oestrogen replacement therapy will almost always give you a better quality of life, reducing the troublesome symptoms such as vaginal changes or night sweats, and it will certainly help to protect you from heart attack, Alzheimer's and osteoporosis. A gel or patch is as effective as a pill but is easier for the body to use and has fewer side effects.

Your nurse or doctor should also check your weight, height and waist measurement, since this gives a very accurate picture of your personal risk for many diseases.

To doctors and scientists, it's a great concern that being overweight/obese has become 'normal' in the so-called civilised world. Men and women of all ages walk around with rolls of fatty flesh hanging around the middle and thighs and will deny they are obese. Doctors are urged to avoid using the words fat, or obese, or overweight'. The truth is that it is a massive problem and the NHS is already unable to cope financially with the other disabling health issues caused by it.

Fat cells are able to produce oestrogen; so even when your ovaries have stopped producing eggs and their chemical messengers have stopped asking your body to produce oestrogen, the fat around your midriff can continue to produce some. This is partly why so many women who are overweight have lovely skin well into their 50's, they also have a high risk of type 2 diabetes and breast cancer.

Why breast cancer? All of the studies into the safety of hormone replacement therapy tell us that the longer a woman has oestrogen in her body, the higher her chance of developing breast cancer. So, to reduce your chances of developing breast cancer, lean and fit is the body you will be aiming for. The number of new patients being diagnosed with type 2 diabetes is shocking doctors and scientists, and it is likely that at any time there are over 100,000 people in UK alone who are not yet diagnosed.

If you know someone who has had type 2 diabetes, then you'll know that it isn't a simple disease. The long-term effects of being insulin resistant, so that your body is unable to manage the glucose (sugar) in your body, are severe and horrible.

Many patients eventually have to use a daily and sometimes two and three times daily, injection of insulin. If you are unable to reduce the amount of sugar in your body by diet and exercise, then by the time of menopause you may already have problems with sensitivity in your feet, and you'll certainly notice sweet smelling urine.

How can you measure yourself to know if you're obese or overweight? Weighing yourself and measuring your height will give you a good idea of BMI or body mass index. This is the usual measurement used within the medical profession.

Waist measurement is also a really good indicator of obesity, so, regardless of your height or build, for most adults a waist measurement of greater than **94 cm** for men and **80 cm** for women is an indicator of the level of internal fat deposits which coat the heart, kidneys, liver, digestive organs and pancreas. This can increase the risk of heart disease, type 2 diabetes and stroke.

What is my BMI? You can work out your BMI by using a calculator, chart or using the formula below. To calculate your BMI, you'll need to know your weight in kilos and your height in metres, then follow the example below:

Step One: multiply your height in metres by itself, eg. 1.7 x 1.7 =2.89

Step Two: divide your weight in kilos by this figure, eg. 80 divided by 2.89 = 27.7

Step Three: for this example, 27.7 is your BMI

See also the chart below to use your BMI and check if you are a healthy weight for your height.

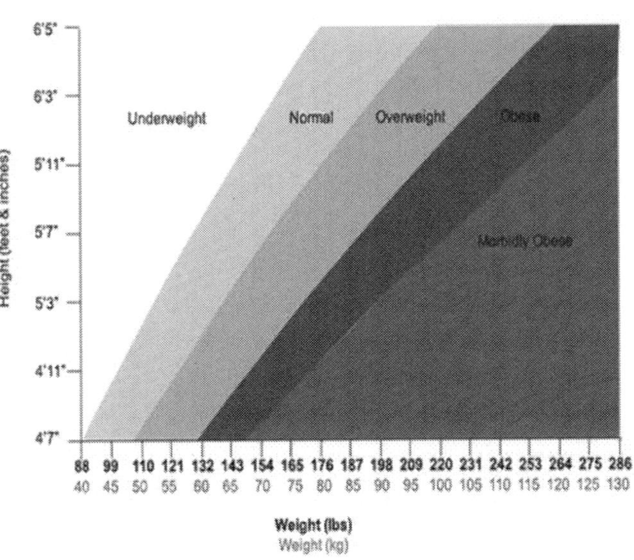
Height (feet & inches)
6'5"
6'3"
5'11"
5'7"
5'3"
4'11"
4'7"
Underweight
Normal
Overweight
Obese
Morbidly Obese
88 99 110 121 132 143 154 165 176 187 198 209 220 231 242 253 264 275 286
40 45 50 55 60 65 70 75 80 85 90 95 100 105 110 115 120 125 130
Weight (lbs)
Weight (kg)

TREATMENTS / REMEDIES

Many women put off going to see their doctor with symptoms of menopause because they feel that the doctor won't have time to listen to them and, in the end, all the doctor will offer is a prescription for HRT or anti-depressant.

I've written this book to empower you to make informed decisions regarding your own menopause, so that if a doctor offers you a prescription for something you don't want to take, you can have a good and reasonable discussion about alternatives. Then you can design a treatment plan together to suit you, not the National Health or your insurance company.

I'm also going to give you some words to use which should guarantee that your doctor not only listens to but understands your concerns, and the words which will ensure you get a prescription for the very latest and best treatment options available today.

In this chapter I'm going to cover current treatments available in UK and Europe which will be similar to what is available in most countries. I'll be including alternative, complementary treatments and prescription medications. There is ongoing research into new evidence-based treatments which may become available in the next two to three years. I hope to update this chapter when they become available. Don't wait until the symptoms become unbearable and you feel that you're losing your mind, make an appointment with your doctor or nurse and talk to them. You don't have to leave with a prescription. When your body is going through early and mid-stage menopause you will most likely just feel that *you want your old self back to be able to live your life well and in control.* If you say nothing else to your doctor, say that.

Everyone's Menopause is different, so don't listen to other people who tell you that you *should* be doing this or taking that, let them have their own experiences and results; but in order to have the best experience for yourself, you need to understand more about it.

Live your menopause your way and don't let anyone else's experience encourage you to feel any different. Only you and your supporting doctor or nurse should be deciding how you're going to deal with it.

10-20% of women are really lucky and report no symptoms of menopause at all, but most women do have symptoms and most of those women have symptoms which interfere with the quality of their lives. If you are taking combined contraception therapy when your body begins perimenopause, then your symptoms might be more manageable, if you notice them at all. However, once you reach 50 or 51 and your doctor takes you off contraception hormones, you may notice symptoms and choose to continue with hormone therapy or try to manage yourself.

The word 'treatment' is not accurate here, although I've used it because it's appropriate. Treatment suggests that there is some problem which needs to be cured, but menopause isn't a disorder or a disease, it's a natural physical process. Maybe the word remedy would be a better choice for the options available to improve the symptoms of menopause.

Here are some quotes from ladies who responded to my questions about their own menopause management.

'*I'm trying to achieve it naturally. I have no idea if I will be able to as I am at the beginning of a journey and nobody knows how long it will last or how much worse my symptoms will get. I'm taking supplements and eating well, I do yoga and meditation but it's tough, really tough. I am on day 61 without a period currently which is the longest I've gone without one (apart from pregnancy) I would never say never to HRT or medical help, I'm taking it day to day. We are all paddling our own canoes and should do what is right for us and our own bodies and minds.'*

'For me it's HRT, tried the natural way for 5 or so years but symptoms were horrendous so my GP suggested that I go on HRT and it suits me, but there is nothing wrong with either way it depending on one's symptoms it's personal preference'

"at 52 it was only this year things started to change for me, had regular periods all my life, missed my first one in April then June none in Aug either.... crazy hot flashes and sleepless nights have started in the last few months... the periods I have had in the last six months are crazy awful, ... So, for me menopause has started. I have always been of the opinion that menopause was completely natural... And when my time came, I would take a vitamin and just ride the storm...... I have always been thankfully healthy, I eat plant based, exercise, don't smoke and I tend, to stay clear of medicines even paracetamol for headaches... Lol... I can cope with the hot flashes, but the sleeplessness is starting to get to me, I really didn't know about the benefits of supplementing oestrogen... In post menopause BUT here is the thing I am absolutely terrified of side effects don't want an animal product (pregnant mares' urine) and worry about the cancer link I have read about, ... I genuinely am so afraid of the long term and possible negative effects of oestrogen., in our home growing up... such subjects would never to spoken about'

The final quote seems typical of the struggle that many women are going through regarding how to manage their menopause. She is saying that she's terrified of the side effects and possible negative effects of adding oestrogen into her body in any way, yet she really hasn't been given much up to date information to make the best decision for herself. This lady needs education on the support and remedies available.

Whichever way you choose to go with regard to prescription medicines, you do need to visit your doctor to see exactly what stage of menopause you're at. If you can, book a double appointment, because doctors don't have a lot of time scheduled for each patient and you want to know that you can have a decent discussion.

This chapter is about all of the options open to you for relief of symptoms of the menopause, looking at complementary therapies, health food supplements, herbal preparations and standard hormone supplements all of which are available in UK and Europe.

Hormone therapy isn't right for all women, for a number of reasons, and the same hormone treatment won't work for everyone. It's a case of educating yourself to understand what remedies are available and then having a discussion with your doctor to see which of those options are possible for you.

I hope you find a team of supporters to help you through these ten years or more, it doesn't matter who is in the team, but feel free to eject anyone who wants to tell you what you should or shouldn't do or take, because you are the Captain of your Team Menopause.

Why is it that so many women are quite happy to use contraception to avoid unplanned pregnancy, but as soon as menopause symptoms make themselves known, they begin to say that they don't want to take HRT because they don't want to put 'chemicals' into their bodies?

Let me explain a little to you about chemicals in medicine (complementary and prescribed) – here's the science – a chemical is an element found within a plant which, when it's introduced to our physical bodies, it causes an effect which creates a response which is either a desired or an undesired response. Thus, it becomes a drug. How chemicals do that isn't for this book, but that is what happens.

So, whether you ingest something from a health food store or from a medical prescription, whether you rub or soak or inhale, you are intending to get a response from the chemical you're using.

In the matter of menopause, the hormones you want to replace, or increase are called oestrogen, testosterone and progesterone which are the chemicals that send messages to your body to increase this or that, or decrease this or that, depending on what's needed. Your entire body runs on a 'feedback system' which is governed by these chemical messengers and that feedback system keeps our bodies running like 'well-oiled machines'. Of course, until the chemical messengers which are also called hormones, stop working in balance with each other; for example, during menopause.

In my own body I produce very little thyroxin from my thyroid gland and that has many consequences which, if left untreated, will result in the death of my body. I take a daily dose of thyroxin hormone – the level required is checked every year. Because of that substituted thyroxin my body behaves the way it was designed to and I get on with my life.

MEDICAL vs ANECDOTAL EVIDENCE: before I list and discuss all remedies available, let me first explain a vital difference or distinction between them.

There are remedies which have strong medical evidence to support their use. In the UK, those remedies are likely to be the only ones a doctor can recommend, and the NHS will pay for. The remedies which have strong medical evidence are approved by the NHS because that evidence is gathered by clinical trials.

Those trials will have involved thousands of women and will always have tested a single pill or therapy either against a placebo (or 'empty sugar' pill or 'empty' therapy) or against the current best-known combination of treatments. These trials often last for several months and usually a year or longer and are monitored. The participants all being interviewed regularly, usually monthly, throughout the trial to discover positive and negative effects of the treatments involved.

After the trial the evidence has to be published and be open to critical discussion by expert doctors and scientists, before the remedy is approved for use within the therapy area it is designed to be used.

Then there is anecdotal evidence where a person uses a product and feels a bit better after use, tells someone else about their experience and causes other people to try the product or therapy. It's a type of hearsay or Chinese whisper but has no base in fact or proof of its effectiveness, simply one person passing on their own findings.

The consumer market for herbal food supplements is hugely profitable for the manufacturers, and sales of single plant extracts or combination pills or powders is currently more than £470 million annually, in the UK alone. Anecdotal evidence has created a health food supplement market around the world. It is often called 'alternative health' and sometimes mistakenly called 'holistic therapy'.

The best option of complementary therapy involves a qualified practitioner taking detailed medical history and looking at your body as a whole instead of each symptom individually. You might find a dietician or nutrition expert, or an herbalist who will suggest and sell you remedies or treatments, and if you feel better and your symptoms are improved then that's a great result.

However, the vast majority of supplements and treatments have no clinical evidence to support the cost of them when they are used to relieve the symptoms of perimenopause and menopause.

Placebo effect: often discussed and never fully explained. It goes along the lines of giving a human a remedy which contains no beneficial ingredients. Not knowing the remedy has no beneficial ingredients humans will usually say they feel better because that's what humans usually do. If you give an animal a remedy which has no beneficial ingredients, the animal will not pretend to be better in order to make you feel good.

There was an interesting experiment carried out last year by the team who make a British TV series called 'Trust Me, I'm a Doctor'. 74 people of both sexes and differing ages and sizes who all had painful knees and had difficulty in walking. They were divided into two groups; the first group being taught exercises to strengthen the muscles supporting the knee joint, the second group were taught the exercises and given a daily pill (they didn't know what was in the pill). All participants were asked to score the level of pain they felt from 1-10 before the experiment began, then score it again after the 8-week trial ended. The results showed that within the group who learned exercises alone, 80% of them reported their

pain had improved by at least 30%. An excellent result. In the group, which was given a pill, 55% of them said their pain had improved by 30%; however, their pill was an empty sugar pill, or placebo.

The most amazing part of this story for me was that in the group being given the placebo supplement, around half of them chose to continue taking it every day, even after being told it was a placebo, *because of the beneficial effect of that pill.* The experiment demonstrates how very effective placebo can be in tricking the mind.

Another trial involved a new anti-depressant medication in which over three thousand people were divided into two groups. One group were given the new pill plus regular sessions with a therapist to discuss their depression and anxiety. The other group were given a placebo plus the sessions with a therapist. At the end of the trial the group taking the anti-depressant showed good improvement in their depression symptoms; the other group also showed good improvement in their symptoms of depression.

However, when the trial ended and they were taken off their placebo pill, the symptoms of depression and anxiety in the second group returned to the pre-trial level, even though both groups continued to have therapy.

It's possible that those women who say they don't want to take HRT because they don't want to put chemicals into their bodies are confused by synthetic vs bioidentical/body identical vs food supplement

COMPOUNDING PHARMACIES: there is a movement, or a trend for clinics to create their own version of a hormonal supplement which, they claim, is unique to each client, and bio-identical to the hormones which the client's own body creates. Well, are they harvesting these hormones from your body and duplicating them in little refrigerated dishes?

No of course not, they're producing hormones from wild yam and soy which mimic the way the hormones produced by your own body behave. The extract of wild yam and soy still have to be processed in a lab and turned into a pill, powder, cream, gel or pessary by adding in other ingredients. They are therefore very similar to the product (produced by regulated companies) and offered by prescription from your doctor.

Those additional ingredients are unregulated, and you won't have any idea of what is actually inside the product you paid for. The cost of this type of 'unique' preparation is high and the safety of the product produced is questionable, since none of those compounding pharmacies need a license and are not regulated.

Their products created especially for you have no evidence of safety since they are being tested only on one person, you. Such compounding pharmacies are not supported by the NHS or medical insurance companies.

BE CAREFUL. There's also a safety issue because some of the creams which are sold and described as containing progesterone, actually don't contain progesterone at a level likely to protect the lining of your womb. This is because it is illegal in the UK to sell a cream with enough progesterone to make a difference to your body. If you supplement your body with oestrogen it will thicken the lining of your uterus and can lead to cancer, so when you still have your uterus, you need to balance the oestrogen with an appropriate dose of progesterone to prevent this thickening.

It isn't that you have to choose between synthetic preparations which have health risks, and expensive bioidenticals only available from private clinics (marketed as all natural and safer) either. As stated elsewhere, there is a long list of preparations available by prescription from your doctor, all made from yam or soy, which mimic your own chemical messengers.

If you don't want to take a prescription from your doctor but want to try to get the same result by yourself, it's possible to buy phytoestrogens, isoflavones and body identical products online. However, there is little research in their effectiveness and safety at unregulated levels.

If you decide to take this route, then at least make sure you buy products which have information and ingredients listed so that you can compare the doses of each ingredient against what you need to get the required result.

I'd like to explain the difference between prescribed medication which will be available only from your licensed health care professional, complementary, and alternative products which are available from many different places - internet, health food shops, complementary practitioners, compounding pharmacies, supermarkets, etc.

Complementary medicine is anything which is used along with medical intervention; alternative medicine is everything used instead of medical intervention.

It is critical for effective health care and consumer protection that practitioners, educators, the industry and regulators, focus on what is important – evidence for safety and effectiveness.

Here there is a clear distinction between substances marketed under the regulations for drugs and those under the far looser regulations for herbs and supplements. Drugs from your doctor or health care provider will typically have far greater evidence for both safety and effectiveness based on the consistent dose prescribed. It will have cost around £450million to develop a medicine to the stage where a doctor prescribes it for a patient. It has had to be trialled on many hundreds, and sometimes thousands, of other people over approximately three years, to make sure that it can: -

- Be safe to use within the limits of what it is prescribed to treat
- Produce a consistent result at the dose it contains
- Cause no harm from the ingredients which take the medicine into the body

And after all of that expense and effort, any medicine can be withdrawn from the market at any time if there are doubts about its safety and efficacy.

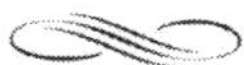

HERBS: and plants that are manufactured and used for medicinal purposes are drugs. They are drugs in the same way that manufactured pharmaceuticals are drugs. A drug is any chemical or combination of chemicals that has biological activity within the body, above and beyond their purely nutritional value. Herbs have little to no nutritional value, but they do contain various chemicals, some with biological activity. Herbs are drugs. The distinction between herbs and pharmaceuticals is therefore a false one.

Herbs are typically marketed based on tradition and anecdote with little scientific evidence for safety or efficacy. While many herbs and plants contain chemical elements, which are very helpful in supporting a healthy human body, you should take care that the dose you buy is adequate to improve the symptom you buy it for.

HORMONE REPLACEMENT THERAPY: or HRT, or hormone supplements. Within the care of women going through menopause, is made up of three main hormones: -

- Progesterone prevents the lining of the womb from thickening; therefore, it protects against cancer of the uterus.
- Testosterone is commonly understood to be a male hormone, but females produce around 3 or 4 times more testosterone than oestrogen before our periods stop. Testosterone is important in a woman to balance mood swings and concentration, for libido or sex drive, energy, bone and muscle strength. Loss of muscle tissue reduces your body's metabolism, leading to low level weight gain unless more exercise is taken.

- Testosterone is supplied as a gel and is massaged into the arm in the same way as an oestrogen gel. Although unlicensed in the UK for women, there are few negative health risks by using testosterone gel, and the benefits, especially in mood and energy supply are welcome if it is appropriate for you.

- Oestrogen has many effects on your body within menopause, such as balance of the vasomotor which causes hot flushes and night sweats, it increases uptake of serotonin which will help to relieve emotional and cognitive functions, and it can increase thickness of skin within your vagina, allowing comfortable intercourse and reducing infection.

The first hormone therapy was created from pregnant horses' urine, which is still prescribed to very many women with no ill effects. The newer products are created from yam and soya, producing a body identical form of oestrogen and progesterone, which means it's the same molecular structure as the hormones your own body can produce.

Supporting your symptoms using prescribed medication is also trial and error because all bodies are unique. However, you get the benefit of discussing your personal risks with a doctor who understands them and what's appropriate for you. Some doctors have developed interest in complementary medicine and may be able to advise you about using herbal supplements along with your normal diet and/or other prescribed medicine.

Starting hormonal therapy by age 50 gives you a reduction in risk of developing osteoporosis, Alzheimer's and heart attack, and although data shows that you can reduce the risk of these diseases even if you don't begin to take oestrogen until age 60, the sooner you start to replace your body's own production of oestrogen the better your long term health will be. This doesn't take into account other benefits of replacing oestrogen which are better quality skin, muscle mass, ability to function well emotionally and physically.

Reasons why you might choose to avoid hormone supplement therapy:

- HRT has been tried but not tolerated (usually because of side effects)
- You choose a more 'natural' approach
- You are worried about negative publicity around HRT

Medical reasons for not using hormone supplement therapy:

- Recent heart attack or poorly controlled angina
- Recent blood clot in the lung or leg
- Active breast, ovarian or womb cancer
- Pregnancy
- Undiagnosed vaginal bleeding
- Newly diagnosed high blood pressure

- Liver disease with abnormal function test results
- Family history of any of the above which needs to be discussed with doctor

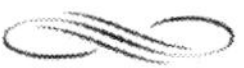

RALOXIFENE: belongs to a class of drugs called SERMS and is licensed for the treatment and prevention of osteoporosis in post-menopausal women. And for lowering the risk of breast cancer in women who are at a high or moderate risk of developing it, due to family history. It is only prescribed for women who have been through the menopause.

It isn't a hormone and will not give any relief to symptoms which are common to the peri menopause or menopause, other than support you physically from the onset of, or increased effects of, osteoporosis. If you have previously fractured a wrist and have a family history of osteoporosis, then this might help you.

TIBOLONE: is an old medication which has a brand name of Livial. It's a prescription medicine and is similar to taking combined HRT in tablet form once daily. It can help relieve symptoms but is not as effective as combined HRT, or an oestrogen with separate progesterone regime. Tibolone is only suitable for post-menopausal women.

ANTI-DEPRESSANTS: none of the anti-depressants prescribed by doctors for the relief of menopausal symptoms (eg hot flushes and night sweats) are licensed to be used this way, but there is anecdotal evidence they might help. Side effects of anti-depressants are (short-term) agitation, anxiety, nausea, lack of interest in life, a feeling of detachment, reduced sex drive and increased appetite. After a few weeks, these side effects should reduce as your body gets used to the drug and, if you have actually been suffering from depression or anxiety not connected to the menopause, then you should be feeling more enthusiastic and calmer about your life. However, many women whose doctors prescribe AD for menopause have found that their anxiety and lack of energy is not helped by them.

CLONIDINE: is a prescription medicine that may help reduce hot flushes and night sweats in some menopausal women. It is not a hormone, it's a synthetic chemical and there is no evidence that it can increase risk of breast cancer. Sadly, it has only a very small effect on menopausal symptoms.

Side effects of clonidine include depression, drowsiness, dry mouth and constipation.

Ultimately, all any of us want to feel is happy; happy that we can live a full and satisfying life, happy that we are loved, happy that we have people in our lives who we love, happy that we have a healthy future, happy that we are safe. That's all, just happy.

EXERCISE: written in bold and capital letters because this does seem to be the thing that all women are able to do for themselves which actually is proven to help relieve many symptoms of menopause. Choose one or several different types of exercise; ones you do by yourself or in a group or in a team and put it on your calendar.

I taught aerobic exercise for around fourteen years and many, many women told me that although they often had to push themselves to attend my class, they always felt much better after it.

Exercise helps with mental health, sleep, general health, weight loss, self-esteem, family life and generally everything. Most importantly, the main long-term health problems created by absence of oestrogen are all improved by doing exercise. Osteoporosis can be avoided by doing regular load-bearing exercise, such as jogging or trampolining or walking (Tena pads are very helpful). Cardiovascular health can be improved by weight loss and aerobic exercise – which can be as little as twenty minutes of moderate paced walking. The risk of stroke is reduced by taking regular moderate exercise.

(My comments are informed by clinical data within internet sites and medical treatment guides. The internet hosts a vast library of clinical trials for every known human disorder. You can easily research by inputting appropriate search words.)

CONVERSATION WITH YOUR DOCTOR

Gynaecological cancer research charity 'The Eve Appeal' has released statistics that highlight the need for better conversation when it comes to women's bodies.

The charity's YouGov research found that 88% of medical professionals think helping patients to express their thoughts or clearly describe their symptoms results in better care and nearly half (47%) agree women not knowing the correct terminology for their reproductive anatomy could lead to delayed diagnosis of a gynaecological cancer.

As well as lack of knowledge regarding the female anatomy, an embarrassment of talking about issues with doctors has been flagged by The Eve Appeal as a reason why some women aren't always opening up when it comes to gynae health.

Women having embarrassment about a physical examination is cited by healthcare professionals as a key factor (51%), followed by embarrassment about how their body looks (39%) and embarrassment talking about gynae issues (37%).

To combat this, The Eve Appeal has launched ***Get Lippy***, a campaign to empower women to having a better understanding of their own bodies and feel comfortable talking to trusted professionals about how to stay healthy.

Here, *Get Lippy* experts share their top tips for talking with your GP about gynae issues so that you can make the most of a short appointment without feeling confused or embarrassed.

1. **KNOW YOUR OWN ANATOMY.** Get clued up on the right vocabulary to explain your problem. It can be difficult for your GP if you refer to your 'bits' or your 'waterworks'. Remember that the vagina is the passage between the uterus and external genitals and the vulva is the external genitals. The new research reveals that nearly half of the healthcare professionals asked to believe that women's lack of female anatomy knowledge could lead to delayed diagnosis of conditions such as womb cancer. Dr Ellie Cannon, an NHS GP, says: "Some gynae symptoms can be vague and hard to describe. A lump in your vagina is very different to a lump on your vulva – make sure you can explain the difference."
2. **THINK AHEAD OF YOUR APPOINTMENT.** What will make you feel more at ease? Don't decline an examination because you've not waxed, shaved or think your vulva doesn't look 'normal' or any other reasons that you may feel are embarrassing. Healthcare professionals don't notice and don't mind, and would always rather you have the examination or screening test you need.
3. **GO ARMED WITH THE CORRECT INFORMATION.** Know your menstrual cycle – and if your periods have stopped, note down when your last period was. Know the name of your contraceptive pill and how long you have been taking it for. Remind yourself of the names of any other medication that you take regularly. Try to be clear in your own mind about when your symptoms started and include all of them. Know when your last cervical screening appointment was – the GP may not have a record if it was done elsewhere. Athena Lamnisos, Chief Executive of The Eve Appeal, says: "Doctors have an average 10 minutes with a patient, and we want to make sure those minutes are well used and that women feel comfortable to talk about their health. We need to get those conversations going and make them count."
4. **DON'T BE AFRAID TO SAY**: Should I be examined / I don't mind being examined. Suggesting it can make for a better consultation and will signal to the GP that you understand that it may be needed and is not a problem for you. Consultant physician and TV doctor

5. Naomi Sutton says: "I want to reassure women there is nothing too embarrassing to consult a doctor or nurse about. We are so used to looking at vulvas and vaginas – please come and talk to us."
6. **DO ASK FOR A FEMALE DOCTOR IF YOU PREFER**, or a double appointment if you think it will give you more time and comfort to be relaxed. If it helps you to bring someone to the appointment with you, this is also fine. Research for The Get Lippy campaign shows that 88% of medical professionals agree that helping patients to express their thoughts or clearly describe their symptoms results in better care.
7. **ASK FOR A DEADLINE**. Know when the doctor wants to follow up if things haven't improved. Gynae symptoms that go on and on must be followed up so ask your doctor when to book a review appointment. Lydia Brain, who was diagnosed with a rare endometrial tumour aged just 24, says: "It took me more than two years to be diagnosed and that's not acceptable. We need to feel confident about talking to medical professionals about our bodies.

ALTERNATIVE/COMPLEMENTARY THERAPY

Paying a professional, qualified alternative or complimentary therapist is often helpful to relieve some of the symptoms of menopause. Acupuncture, aromatherapy, cognitive behavioural therapy, herbal medicine, reflexology, EFT (tapping), nutrition and relaxation therapy are all practiced by people who have taken nationally and internationally recognised qualifications which will reassure you that they are competent in their practice.

If you've decided to try and manage your mood swings and hot flushes without medical intervention, think about what you can do within your lifestyle that might help. For example, exercise of any kind has been proven to provide physical and emotional support. Any exercise, whether by yourself at home or out in nature, in a group class or in the gym/swimming pool. Also cutting down on alcohol, cigarettes and caffeine are strongly recommended.

It is important to note, however, that although any or some of these therapies can be helpful in the management of some symptoms, they will not offer any protection from the long-term problems associated with loss of oestrogen; for example, osteoporosis and cardiovascular health.

If you use any of these therapies, it's important to tell your doctor so that you can include them in your general health treatment plan. Typically, you would visit a therapist/practitioner for any of these treatments once or twice a month, depending on your treatment plan. There is no evidence that any of them will work for everyone, but some can offer help in reducing the number of hot flushes, night sweats, improving the quality of sleep and reducing feelings of anxiety and brain fog. Long term there is no evidence that any of those symptoms will not simply come back as soon as you take a break from the therapy.

However, the relationship you have with your therapist/practitioner can be a huge support at a time when you may be feeling alone and unsupported, isolated and worried about your ability to control your life.

ESSENTIAL OILS: are used in Aromatherapy and will typically involve a visit to a therapist or practitioner who will discuss your symptoms, your family health history and how you live your life. Oils will be mixed for you during your visit, because one mixture will not be right for everyone, and usually it will be applied to you as a massage. By itself, the massage should be comforting and soothing and just being able to switch off and relax for an hour is an enormous benefit.

If you want to try using essential oils at home, here's a list of a few which are helpful during early and later menopause, along with some hints on how to use them yourself. Do take care where you buy these oils from because the quality is important, the label must read PURE ESSENTIAL OIL, otherwise it could be a blend and you have no idea what is in the bottle. NEVER DRINK ESSENTIAL OILS, EVEN DILUTED IN WATER OR ANY OTHER LIQUID, they are not produced to be taken internally and bottles of oil from reputable suppliers will ALWAYS SAY SO ON THE LABEL.

Clary Sage: can be helpful for mental clarity and is a mood balancer. Try two or three drops onto a paper tissue to sniff regularly when you feel mental confusion or overwhelm. You can also keep a bottle of it in the bathroom or your work desk. Using a teaspoon to measure (teaspoon equals 5ml liquid) pour sweet almond oil or jojoba or pure coconut oil (never mineral oil such as baby oil) into a small, clean bottle with a secure lid. For every teaspoon measured, you can add 2 or 3 drops only of essential oil. Keep this bottle cool and in a dark place and the blended contents should be good for a couple of months.

Use it on your feet and rub your lower arms and around your neck during times when you feel a hot flush coming on. You can also use drops of oils in water and add into an electric vaporizer or small bowl over a tea light candle, this produces droplets of the oil in the air you breathe.

Lavender: this is one of the most useful oils, ever. It's the one and only oil which can be used undiluted on your skin (never on broken or grazed skin) Calming and balancing, lavender can be used in any of the ways suggested above. This oil is especially helpful in relaxation and is sleep inducing.

Geranium: this is one of my absolute favourites and is a deeply feminine oil. Comforting and supportive, you could use this oil in a tissue when you feel overwhelmed or anxious. If you blend this (as described above for clary sage) in a bottle to keep with you, add some lavender as well.

Rosemary: brilliant for helping to clear your head when you feel confused or anxious. It's helpful for memory as well and has been on the desk in many academic examination rooms.

Ylang ylang: so great they named it twice. This oil is deeply sedative so is brilliant for inducing sleep and relaxation during meditation or yoga. However, it's also an aphrodisiac, so if your libido is running low (or your partner's) try this dropped onto paper and placed between your pillow and pillowcase. The effect it will have on you will have to be discovered by you, then use it accordingly. BUT, if it makes you drowsy, please don't use it before driving or doing any task which requires you to be alert.

COGNITIVE BEHAVIOURAL THERAPY or CBT: Your doctor may be able to prescribe CBT for you, especially if you are unable to take HRT due to medical reasons. CBT can be really useful in re-framing how you see your life and the stories you tell yourself and others about your life and can be helpful in relieving feelings of stress and anxiety because of those stories and the way you continue to live.

During menopause those stories can overtake your thoughts and be hijacked by the low mood caused by a lack of serotonin. When you're not sleeping well and trying to maintain your usual family and work routines, the lack of serotonin can turn any of those stories into nightmares. If you struggled to make friends in earlier life, then your brain can turn that story into how unlovable and hopeless you are.

Stress can overcome you when there's a situation that seems too difficult or that you haven't had training on, and you don't know where to begin to solve the situation. In your thirties and forties, you managed to resolve those kinds of problems, but when perimenopause begins, you might feel a lack of confidence and inability to achieve a good outcome. CBT may be able to help you with this.

You may have feelings of being unsafe or under threat from normal situations you would usually be able to solve. You know that you feel under threat because your body begins to change as if you were being attacked; breath gets shallow and fast, heart begins to pump faster, your eyes might be brighter, and you begin to feel adrenalin pumping. These are not normal reactions to discovering you left something unfinished in the office, but if you're in perimenopause and short of serotonin, you might be unable to focus on things and feel out of control. CBT can help you with this.

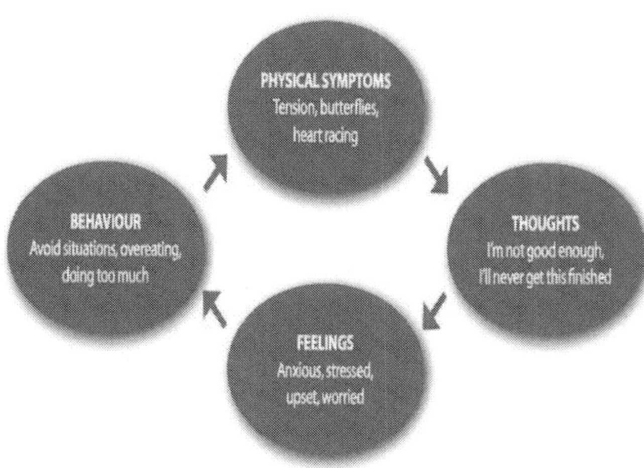

CBT is useful for emotional support from yourself to yourself at times when stress levels rise. Women who underwent CBT training in the hope of hot flush management, found they were experiencing fewer events daily, which also affected the number of night sweats they had. How it works is that you practice self-awareness before, during and after an event, keep a diary or log and make notes of how you felt after each hot flush. Women will say they feel their face is bright red and sweat is pouring off their head and down their breasts. Obviously, this creates feelings of embarrassment and shame, but reality might be that, for the majority of women, a hot flush in the office or workplace isn't nearly as bad as this. Just because you feel others are watching you, the feelings of embarrassment are higher, therefore you are more stressed, therefore the hot flush gets worse. It becomes a self-perpetuating cycle, which you can break when you know how to. We all are able to think a situation is much worse than it is and are able to create shame and embarrassment from thin air. Truthfully, most of your colleagues won't even notice you when you feel a hot flush washing over you, and it's only your actual behaviour which will alert them to something wrong.

HERBAL MEDICINE: herbs and plants used for medicinal purposes are drugs and are as much drugs as any pharmaceutical on prescription. The definition of a drug is any chemical which can create a change within the body but is not nutrition. So, herbs which you buy in order to relieve menopause symptoms are drugs, and any advertising which suggests that they are safer or more organic or natural than pharmaceuticals, is misleading you.

There's a huge difference between working with a qualified herbalist and buying health food supplements from a supermarket or drug store. An herbalist should be registered with the National Institute of Medical Herbalists to be worth paying consultation fees to them.

Here are some herbal supplements which women with mild symptoms have found to be useful. There is no medical or clinical evidence to support a doctor advising you on their use unless he has an interest in herbology, but you can buy any of these over the counter. Many women say they have found relief of menopausal symptoms from herbs, and even if it's only a better night's sleep, it might be worth the cost.

How much you should take: this cannot be answered since there is no clinical evidence to say that the bottle in your hand contains the quantity required to produce the result you need.

What do I mean by that? There are many clinical studies undertaken on the benefit of phytoestrogens and isoflavones extracted from plants and used to replace the oestrogen, progesterone and testosterone which your body no longer produces. Extractions from soy, wild yam, black cohosh or red clover are typically used. While the supplements available to buy will (probably) have been created from herbs and plants, there is no regulation about the quantity of the active ingredient inside the supplement; and, although the marketing of that supplement may say something such as "isoflavones are *clinically proven* to ease symptoms of menopause" you need to look carefully to ensure that the dose inside that pill is the same as the dose used to achieve the result within the clinical trial. How do you discover that? Look it up on the internet is my best advice.

For a manufacturer to make any beneficial medicinal claim for his product, there has to have been some research into the use of that product for the symptom it is sold to relieve. For example, a study could have found that a daily intake of 250mg of EPA and DHA (Omega-3 fatty acids found within oily fish etc.) is beneficial to the normal function of the heart. The bottle you hold in your hand while you browse the shelves mentions on the label that its contents 'may help with the healthy function of the heart', but you don't know what dose is 'helpful' because you didn't read that study; so do you buy it and hope, or find a product that provides full information on its label?

I'm sure you have friends or workmates who tell you they got relief from night sweats by using such and such a brand of wild yam or black cohosh, and that will be true for them, great, but you may not get the same result. Buying a supplement can be trial and error, and ultimately expensive.

It's also important to be aware that if you choose to buy health food supplements to ease your menopause symptoms rather than take a prescription for a similar product because you're worried about the connection with breast cancer and weight gain from prescribed medicine. The active ingredient of isoflavone or phytoestrogens within those food supplements will mimic your own oestrogen in exactly the same way as the prescribed medicine.

There is good clinical evidence to demonstrate that these supplements have the same risk of causing and/or 'feeding' the breast cancer gene which is hormone dependant. To reduce the risk of cancer and weight gain caused by such supplements the manufacturers will often reduce the dose of the active ingredients; that's ok but now you're buying a product which isn't effective at easing the symptoms you bought it for.

Regulation in the UK, we have a system called the Traditional Herbal Registration (THR) which was set up to provide some level of safety for consumers of herbal supplements. Look for the THR logo on the pack or bottle.

While herbal supplements have been used for centuries, there is no guarantee of potency suitable for you. You have absolutely no guarantee of their quality, purity, source or concentration, unless the product comes with a manufacturer's money back guarantee. Some products might interfere with other medication and supplements you already take. The shop assistant will not be able to advise you because they aren't medically trained. St John's Wort, ginseng and grapefruit are all known to reduce and/or increase the effect of some other medications, so discuss the addition of any supplement with your doctor before starting to take it. That doesn't mean that your doctor understands herbal medicine, but they may know about complications.

- **Agnus castus (vitex agnus castus):** it is said that this herb works on the pituitary gland which sends messages to the ovaries to release hormones. Therefore, it's only useful during perimenopause when your body is still producing oestrogen to be released. Some women have reported that it can help with mood swings, anxiety and tension.
- **Black cohosh (cimicifuga racemose):** this is an herb which people who work in a health food store will tell you sells most often for the reduction of hot flushes. There is no clinical evidence to support its use

for the reduction of hot flushes, but some women have found it to be helpful. It is banned in some countries because some strains of the herb have been found to cause liver damage. Always chose a product which is in some way tested and carries an assurance of purity and quality.

- **Red clover**: this has been found to be rich in phytoestrogens which can mimic your own supply of oestrogen, and many women report that it reduces the severity of hot flushes and vaginal dryness. It's one of the most popular herbal supplements in some parts of the world. Up to now, there is no evidence that using red clover will reduce the number or severity of hot flushes or any other symptom of menopause. Because there is no evidence for its use, there can be no safe or effective dose recommended. The use of daily high doses of red clover has been known to cause a vaginal bleed and it can feed hormonally driven cancers, such as breast, uterine, endometrial, ovarian etc. So, if you have any family history of any of these cancers you should speak to your doctor before starting a course of red clover. Red clover causes toxic effects when taken with methotrexate, a drug used to treat certain types of cancer and to control severe psoriasis or rheumatoid arthritis. Tamoxifen is a drug commonly used in the treatment of breast cancer; red clover interacts with tamoxifen and can reduce the medical effects of tamoxifen. Speak to your doctor before using red clover. It will also interact and reduce the effectiveness or create a dangerous combination with commonly used drugs such as anti-depressants and PPIs such as lansoprazole or omeprazole. Most especially, red clover can have a negative effect on anti- coagulants such as warfarin, clopidogrel, dalteparin and others.
- **CBD oil**: a newcomer to the choice of supplements is cannabidioil. It's the essential oil of the flax/hemp plant and is often confused with cannabis/marijuana. It is illegal to sell any hemp/flax product in Europe which has any more than 0.2% THC content. It's the THC which causes a feeling of euphoria, or the psychoactive 'high' which cannabis users look for and which is often addictive. Therefore, regulated CBD oil sold within Europe should never cause the user to experience any heightened mental state. Many women have found that this oil is helpful in relieving symptoms of the menopause as well as depression, anxiety, sleep problems and a general balancing of the body systems. Again, it's important that you speak to your doctor before you start taking this because there may be complications around other

medications that you take. Your doctor is very unlikely to know any more than you do about its effects on other medications, so ask the person who supplied your CBDoil to explain the use and 'dose' to you. Do your research, look up on the internet as much as you can find about it. There is some concern about the use or overuse of CBD oil in patients who are taking other medications which are sometimes lifesaving. Chemotherapy for example, can be less effective if the patient also takes CBDoil. It's vital that if you are taking other medications, you discuss this with your doctor.

- **Flax:** as the older sister of CBD oil, the benefits of using cold-pressed flax oil are well known. It is a rich source of phytoestrogens which can mimic your body's own oestrogen activity. Relief from hot flushes or sleep disturbance is the usual benefit claimed. I use virgin flax oil as a dressing on my salad, you should never heat up a cold pressed oil since the magic is within its cold fresh state.
- **St John's Wort:** has been shown to help with mood swings and feelings of depression, but there is no evidence that it can help with hot flushes or night sweats. Most importantly, you should consult your doctor before using it because it can interfere with other medications, especially anti-depressants.

It's also worth noting that because your body has such a thorough feedback system of keeping itself working well, any excess number of vitamins or minerals or other supplements will be excreted from the body in urine or stools.

The North American Menopause Society or NAMS brought together a team of experts to take a critical look at all the available studies on herbs, supplements, and other nonhormonal approaches for treating hot flushes.

What did they find? They found that besides maybe soy foods and soy supplements, no other herb or supplement showed an effect any greater than a sugar pill (placebo). Soy did get a qualified nod from the team because it may help some women, but only those women whose bodies can use soy to produce a compound called equol, often those women of Asian descent. An equol supplement that may help other women is being developed, but it's not on the market yet.

You can buy body cream containing extract of wild yam in many places, but those creams often don't contain yam and sometimes they've been adulterated with steroids, including oestrogen and progesterone type compounds. See Resources secion for NAMS website.

BE AWARE: some products should carry a warning triangle as they have been proven to be either ineffective or actually unsafe. Including:

- Evening primrose oil, it can interfere with other medication
- Ginseng can cause vaginal bleeding and is ineffective for hot flushes
- Vitamin E in high doses can be very dangerous and does nothing for menopausal symptoms
- Red clover in high doses can cause uterine bleed

Reasons why you might choose to avoid hormone supplement therapy:

- HRT IS medically unadvisable
- HRT has been tried but not tolerated (usually because of side effects)
- You choose a more 'natural' approach
- You are worried about negative publicity around HRT

Medical reasons for not using hormone supplement therapy:

- Recent heart attack or poorly controlled angina
- Recent blood clot in the lung or leg
- Active breast or womb cancer
- Pregnancy
- Undiagnosed vaginal bleeding
- Newly diagnosed high blood pressure
- Liver disease with abnormal function test results
- Family history of any of the above which needs to be discussed with doctor

NUTRITION: Outside of taking modern body-identical hormones prescribed by a doctor, I've read the largest number of success stories from women who persevere and succeed using good nutrition and exercise programmes. These success stories come from women managing their symptoms of menopause well, and who are able to get on with their lives.

A good nutritionist will give personal advice on how diet and lifestyle affect hormone function and will recommend the right amounts of the right foods for you to eat in order to stay healthy.

I've read some strong anecdotal evidence that a diet rich in soy-based foodstuffs can be helpful to lessen the number and strength of hot flushes, and to improve mood and general feelings of well-being.

There are several elements which are often missing or in low supply in women around the age of menopause. Increasing these as needed and adding in some other foodstuffs appears to have created the successes mentioned above.

Iron: a lack of iron can cause general fatigue, loss of hair and brittle nails.

Vitamin B: the vitamin B family is responsible for general good health, especially the nervous system, energy, mental health.

Magnesium: this is responsible for good bone, muscle and nerve function.

Calcium: very necessary for strong bone health.

Essential fatty acids: we have been told for years that EFAs are an essential part of heart health but are often forgotten when weight management is an issue.

Obviously, these are only a few elements of a good diet which can improve menopausal symptoms and you can find out more from any number of books or internet sites or find a local nutritionist and build a great relationship.

HORMONE SUPPLEMENT THERAPY

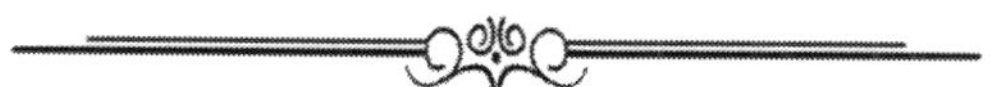

Around the turn of the 21st century a study was conducted called the Jubilee which questioned 200 women aged between 50 and 64 about their lives before and after menopause. Surprisingly, 65% were happier than before menopause began, 66% had greater independence, and 59% said their relationships were better. 48% said their working lives had improved after menopause and only 15% said their work performance and status had deteriorated.

There were differences among those women who were taking HRT and those who were not. 50% of those on HRT reported an improvement in their sex lives, compared to only 18% of those not taking it.

Almost 67% taking HRT said their working lives were improved and they were able to pursue their career track, compared to 56% of those not on HRT.

In general, 71% of women taking HRT said their general health and wellbeing had improved, compared to 48% of those not taking it. At the end of 2019 over 13 million women in UK are menopausal or post-menopausal, yet only one million are taking HRT.

HRT or hormone supplements shouldn't be seen as magic bullets which take away all pain and those who are on them can hover above the ground while peeing champagne. No, that isn't the case. This type of medication does not suit everyone, and not everyone is able (for various medical reasons) to even try it.

You have to be prepared to be patient and if the first type you try doesn't suit you, then go back to the doctor and have further discussion about other types. Different doses and different methods of application could be tried. It's worth sticking with it and reaching a solution, which may take several tries, because you could end up 'hormone-rich and happy' and that isn't a bad thing.

Interestingly, while those in the Jubilee study who were taking HRT were given the group nickname of HRH or hormone-rich and happy, that group had the greatest weight gain in their post menopause years; but were still able to demonstrate a truly positive outlook and more vitality.

Your priority should be in getting the best treatment to suit yourself from your doctor, whether or not that includes a prescription for hormone supplements or anti-depressants. This is why this book will help your discussion and arm you with information which will allow you and your doctor to explore the best plan for you. Going to your doctor doesn't mean that you have to take hormone supplements if you choose not to; but it does mean that your doctor is able to provide you with continuing care while you live through this transition.

In 2015 the UK body which decides which medicines can and cannot be provided to patients by the NHS published guidelines on how to manage women in perimenopause and menopause. The UK body is called NICE or the National Institute for Clinical Evidence. It's disappointing that, 4 years later, the average family doctor in the UK has little knowledge of those guidelines. Thankfully, the medical profession is trying to catch up quickly since menopause is being discussed by public figures in the media, every day, and currently there are record numbers of women visiting their doctors to talk about their symptoms. The guidelines are updated regularly, and the most recent update was published in December 2019. It can be found at http://pathways.nice.org.uk/pathways/menopause. One reason why your doctor might seem unsure about a diagnosis is that peri menopause and menopause have such a broad range of symptoms.

As previously stated, oestrogen affects all of your body in some way because it is a chemical messenger within your body's feedback system. Therefore, during a busy surgery your doctor might struggle to understand the symptoms you present with, and not connect the dots between your age and those symptoms.

However, there are some reasons why you might not have the best possible outcome from a visit to your GP. These reasons are often outside of your own doctor's control because he is employed by the NHS, he is expected to prescribe what he has been told to, even if that isn't exactly what his patient has asked for. That sounds a little convoluted, so let me explain a bit more.

In the UK, all of our family doctors are employed in medical centres or health centres, and all those places are governed by a group called a local Clinical Commissioning Group, or CCG. This CCG is responsible for the spending of the taxpayer's pound and will have an approved list (a formulary) of everything a doctor or nurse is able to prescribe to patients, over every area of medicine.

There are many areas of the UK where the list of products which are licensed to be prescribed for use by women to relieve the symptoms of menopause hasn't been updated by the local CCG for years. The reasons for that aren't known to me. What that means to you is that although you might have a good relationship with your doctor and your doctor understands your need for a specific item, if the local CCG does not want that specific item to be prescribed, your doctor will receive a 'warning' on his computer. Your doctor will then need to justify why the item is prescribed.

The good news is that if the item your doctor is trying to prescribe for you is appropriate for your health care, and if the item is in line with current NICE guidance, your doctor can prescribe a medication which is not on his local formulary, but which he can justify prescribing.

If you are fortunate to live anywhere in the UK then your visits to the doctor or nurse are free, unlike anywhere else in the world. In Europe every visit to a doctor costs between Euro 20-50 and is paid when the appointment is made, to be reclaimed from health insurance later, if you have it.

In the last 12-15 years the pharmaceutical industry has been busy researching and developing more body identical supplements made from wild yam and soy. These are very much more acceptable to the human body and have the same chemical structure as your own hormones, which means they are easier to metabolise and produce fewer unwanted side effects. They also mimic your natural oestrogen and progestogen almost exactly.

These supplements are available in pill, patches, gel, vaginal pessaries, and vaginal ring. Many of them are licensed (by the body which governs medicine in your country), to be used where "the relief of post-menopausal symptoms is required in cases where those symptoms **SIGNIFICANTLY REDUCE QUALITY OF LIFE"**. Remember what I said about the magic phrase to use in discussion with your doctor? That's it. Some of them are available at any stage of the menopause but use those words anyway.

The original hormone supplements available to women suffering from symptoms of menopause were created from pregnant mare's urine. Those products are still available, often used but no longer first choice today. They were useful and for the first time, women had some hope of being free from the more brutal symptoms of menopause. Side effects are the main problem with them though, because they are far from being similar to our own oestrogen in chemical makeup.

Body identical supplements are not only available to those who can pay to go private, the British NHS has a list of them which can be prescribed, and the same is true in Europe and many other countries. These include (NB: the same product can be called other names in different parts of the world) Oestrogel, (a gel with two strengths of oestrogen from soy or yam), Utrogestan (progesterone from yam) and a vaginal oestrogen called Vagifem (from soy or yam), or there's topical Ovestin cream (from yam).

There is a myth that taking a hormone supplement only masks the symptoms of menopause and 'you have to go through it (menopause) sometime'. I've heard this said many times, and the truth is that no woman knows how long her symptoms will last, which is why there's no upper age limit for taking hormone supplement. Remember that if you make the decision to stop taking it, you need to discuss this with your doctor and agree a withdrawal plan so that your symptoms don't come crashing back in a 'whiplash' kind of effect.

Relationships within family and work can get stretched to breaking if your menopausal symptoms are really getting in your way. Whatever you choose to do about managing yourself within the peri and menopause, bear in mind that you're not going through it in isolation and many others are being affected daily by your decisions.

Reasons why you might choose not to take hormone supplement therapy:

- HRT IS medically unadvisable
- HRT has been tried but not tolerated (usually because of side effects)
- You choose a more 'natural' approach
- You are worried about negative publicity around HRT

Reasons why you should not take hormone supplements are very few, but doctors are aware of these and with a change of application or dosage some of these reasons are obsolete:

- History of stroke or TIA
- Pregnancy
- Recent heart attack or poorly controlled angina
- History of blood clot (although using a gel or cream is safe)
- High risk endometrial cancer
- Active breast cancer or family history of
- Unexplained vaginal bleeding (not menstrual)
- Active liver disease
- Newly diagnosed high blood pressure

Just because it's the most effective treatment for symptoms of menopause doesn't mean hormone supplement therapy has to be 'YOUR' treatment of choice.

If you have a uterus you also need to add in micronized progesterone (the safest and all natural); if you have had a hysterectomy, then you don't need progesterone. Any side effects experienced on one type of progesterone might be relieved by changing the brand or method of administration.

Last year new trials were published at the San Antonio Breast Cancer Symposium in Texas. The findings from those trials are that taking oestrogen alone reduces the risk of a patient developing breast cancer by 23%. If you've had a hysterectomy for whatever reason, this should encourage you to discuss hormone therapy treatment for your menopause.

Progesterone supplement in perimenopause isn't necessary if you already use a uterine coil, since that coil contains and slowly releases, a synthetic progestin.

If you start taking hormone supplements in the early part of your perimenopause, when you still have fairly regular periods, you may be offered sequential HRT which means that the progestogen is taken for 10-14 days every month and the oestrogen taken every day. As your own oestrogen depletes, and your periods come less frequently, your progestogen can be taken for only 2 weeks out of every 3 months; this is called long cycle HRT and is always a 3-month cycle.

Evidence shows that by replacing the oestrogen, which your body no longer produces, you will protect your blood vessels and cardiovascular system which reduces the risk of heart attack and stroke – number one cause of death of women in UK. Hormone supplement therapy can also:

- Improve bone density, loss of oestrogen is the number one risk factor for developing osteoporosis
- Reduce cholesterol, high LDL cholesterol is a strong risk factor for heart disease
- Will reduce your chance of developing type 2 diabetes so long as your diet is healthy
- Recent studies also show that beginning to replace oestrogen early can protect against development of dementia and Alzheimer's disease.

In **post menopause** (when your periods have been absent for 12 months or you're aged 54 or older), progestogen can be taken every day along with the oestrogen to produce continuous combined HRT, which means you have no bleed at all. Except for the first 6 months on this routine, during which you may experience some light bleeding, which you should discuss with your doctor. Both of these hormones will be prescribed at the lowest dose and titrated up if necessary. Your doctor will best advise you here and not every woman will get the same advice because we're all different.

Whenever you start a course of any type of hormone therapy, at whatever stage of your life, and for whatever reason, there will be a delay between beginning the medication and feeling the results. Occasionally there will be side effects which you cannot tolerate, and you should make a note of how you're feeling as the weeks go by. Don't give up though, because there will be an alternate product or method of use that will suit you.

Side effects of hormonal supplements include: -

- Headaches
- Swollen or tender breasts
- Bloating
- Swelling in other parts of the body
- Indigestion or changes in bowel movements
- Vaginal bleeding or spotting
- Leg cramps
- Nausea

In other words, much the same as when you began to use hormonal contraception.

Within hormone therapy for the menopause, doctors advise a three-month period on the same supplement to see how it works for you. You will have visited your doctor or health clinic in the first place because you were experiencing symptoms that were getting in your way and causing you to avoid some situations or stop some activities. It's a good idea to write those symptoms in a journal and, during this period of time while your body gets used to the supplement, jot down if there is any alteration in the symptom; is it better or worse?

After three months, if you don't feel that you have relief from those symptoms or you don't like the side effects, then you and your doctor can try a different dosage or a different supplement altogether. Maybe go to a gel instead of patch, or just switch a brand, because not all supplements will behave the same way for everyone.

You can continue to use hormone therapy for the rest of your life if you want to. Regular health checks will ensure you stay fit and well and the level of hormone therapy should be reduced as you get older. There is no reason for a doctor to tell you to stop taking it if you feel well and have no health risk.

When you decide to stop using hormone therapy you should have that discussion with your doctor and make a plan for a gentle and slow reduction of your medication. Stopping hormone supplements abruptly can cause a 'whiplash' effect of symptoms and you might think your menopause has come back again. This is unlikely to happen.

Safety of Hormone Supplements: when I was going through menopause the Women's Health Initiative (WHI) study had just been published which gave an impression that women who took oral HRT were at much greater risk of developing breast cancer than women who did not.

This one statement changed the way women were treated for around 17 years; I was one of the thousands of casualties of that study because my doctor advised me to stop taking my hormone supplements. Unfortunately, the information used from that study not only withdrew access to a group of truly helpful and life enhancing therapies, but it left most younger women scared out of using the most effective therapy for menopause symptoms, when it was their turn.

Following years of analysis of how that study (WHI)was set up and managed, we now know that taking hormone supplements during menopause, while not totally risk-free, gives a far smaller risk for breast cancer than a regular pattern of drinking alcohol, and a massively smaller risk for breast cancer than being overweight will give.

However, just like the sensational claims made around children's MMR vaccine and autism, it's very difficult to clear up this kind of false information once people have decided that it's true. I'm always surprised by how contrary us adults are when it comes to deciding what we choose to believe, in spite of evidence for and against our choice.

In essence, what this inaccurate evidence from the WHI study has created is a long period of time when women who should have been able to sail through their menopause, have been left to the whim of the food supplement industry, which has made billions of dollars and euros and pounds of profit by creating hugely successful marketing campaigns for many 'composite' herbal supplements which might or might not have any effect on symptoms they claim to relieve.

Slowly but surely confidence is returning to the use of hormone therapy in peri and post menopause, assisted by the pharmaceutical industry's research and development of safe and effective products.

Post menopause: if you reached early 50s without noticing any symptoms that were a challenge (first of all, lucky you) it's possible that now you are post-menopausal, other symptoms are being noticed and you may feel a need for support. There is a general rule that you can safely begin to take hormone supplement therapy up to 10 years after your last period. So do go and speak to your doctor if you find your symptoms getting worse in post menopause.

Testosterone: females produce around 3 or 4 times the amount of testosterone as they do oestrogen, the production of both decreases through your lifespan. You need testosterone to maintain muscle and bone strength, urogenital health, metabolic function; adequate supply also maintains your cognitive functions. So, when your supply drops, you'll notice a decline in your ability to maintain your usual level of mood, intellectual thought, rational, reasoning, etc. (menopause mind?)

More importantly, if you have a happy and loving relationship, a lack of it can lead to low libido which you'll notice as a loss of sexual desire, arousal and ability to reach orgasm. We've discussed low libido within the chapter titled Sex in Menopause, but if you add in the shortage of testosterone then the problem is explained a little more.

Many women with low testosterone complain of tiredness, as though someone pulled the plug on their vitality supply, that overwhelming weariness means you just want to lie and sleep, anywhere.

When you finally go through menopause, the general lack of balance between oestrogen and testosterone can cause you to develop acne, increased facial hair and male pattern baldness. Some of these symptoms are genetic, so next time you have a family get together, or bring out the old family photograph albums, check out your female relatives.

There are no testosterone medical preparations in the UK which are licensed for use by women; however, if your symptoms are significantly reducing the quality of your life at home or at work, then your doctor is able to prescribe a supplement in the form of a gel.

Possible side effects of testosterone: all women have variable responses to this supplement and for some women, it doesn't suit them at all, or help with their symptoms. Hopefully, with further education, doctors will become more confident about prescribing it and its appropriate dosage.

There are some not so good effects though, which might be because of the dose, so if you develop any of these go back and talk to your doctor, instead of immediately stopping application.

- Increased body hair where you usually apply it – you could spread it more thinly or reduce dose
- More general increased body hair (uncommon)
- Male pattern baldness (uncommon)
- Acne and greasy skin (uncommon)
- Deepening of voice (rare)
- Enlarged clitoris (rare)

Avoid taking a testosterone supplement if you: -

- Are pregnant or breastfeeding
- Have active liver disease
- Have a history of hormone sensitive breast cancer

- Competitive athletes – care must be taken to maintain levels well within the female physiological range

How long can you continue with hormone supplements? There is no maximum time period but women who begin to replace oestrogen early should continue until at least age 51 when periods cease. However, it's also known that staying on hormone replacement therapy until the age of 60 provides women with far more benefits to the whole body than the health risks which may be created by taking it. Many women will stay on HRT after the age of 60 because they like the extra health protection it offers, and they really enjoy the continued feeling of energetic wellbeing.

By the way, stopping treatment with HRT may mean that symptoms will flare again. This doesn't mean that HRT has simply 'masked' your menopause and as soon as you stop it then all the symptoms come back. What it means is that your symptoms were always going to continue for that long anyway and HRT has managed those symptoms until you stop taking it. You should always reduce your dose gradually before stopping and should discuss this with your doctor.

GODDESS ACADEMY

GODDESS ACADEMY

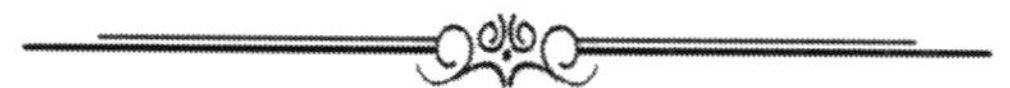

"The best years of your life are the ones in which you decide your problems are your own. You do not blame your mother, the economy, or your boss. You realise that you control your own destiny." Albert Ellis

Ok, so now you're post menopause and beyond the controlling tyranny of hormonal fluctuations. If you've been wearing one, it's time to shed your cloak of menopause misery. You have access to the golden honey pot of the rest of your life.

If you choose to, you could use this period of time to re-invent yourself. Many things will change in your life because of menopause and, for some women, choosing to deliberately change parts of their lives gives a feeling of control and empowerment. We're supposed to grow and change through the years of our lives and if we're not growing then we're dying – just look at a flower.

The end of fertility is not the end of femininity; I know I said that before but I'm saying it again because it really matters. If you've put on a few pounds and your hair has thinned a bit, maybe you notice more wrinkles and find a few whiskers around your mouth; it's possible you might be feeling a bit fed up and not very attractive. Not to diminish all those feelings, but you're not alone.

Don't grieve the end of your fertile years – menopause is your Gateway to Freedom ladies, so pull on your big girl pants (with or without a Tena pad) and walk boldly forward with a smile, into your magnificent maturity. Your future is waiting for you to celebrate the joy of the rest of your life.

The secret to living well and longer is eat half, walk double, laugh triple and love without measure. A Tibetan proverb

Resilience – I offered to tell you why I'm often a figure of inspiration within a community of high achievers and I can sum this up with one word – resilience – that isn't what others see though; they see a woman of vitality and light, a smile and a bounce when she walks, they see confidence. Some people call it grit, tenacity, perseverance, endurance. It doesn't matter which word you choose, what it means to me is that I will not be defeated for very long. The dictionary tells me that the word resilience means the ability to overcome adversity, and I've had plenty of practice at that.

If there is something you really want to do, don't give up on that dream. When I was young, I had one focus and one goal which was to become an air hostess and fly around the world. In the 1960s I knew no-one who had been in an airplane outside of the war and none of my schoolfriends had this dream, so I truly don't know what was driving that ambition. I researched what qualifications I needed to get the position, and all the things I did with my life, from age 16 to 21, were done to give me the experience required.

But it wasn't easy – in the early 1970s being part of an airline was about the most prestigious and glamorous work a girl could get, so competition was strong for every vacancy. The first airline I interviewed for was called Pan Am, (long since closed down) their offices were in Grosvenor Square London. At the age of 21, I was a lumpy and self-conscious girl and owned only one dress. As I walked into the room where all applicants were gathered, I really wanted to turn around and go back to 'hometown'. Dozens of really beautiful girls from Spain, France, Italy who had all flown in just for this interview. I felt outfaced and totally tongue tied. I didn't perform well and wasn't offered a second interview. The next opportunity was with British Caledonian (long since swallowed up by British Airways and the name has gone) whose uniform was tartan. I had given up my job as a hotel receptionist and moved to Manchester where I worked as a 'temp' doing a variety of jobs until I got the big one. British Caledonian had advertised in National newspapers and I applied, qualifications were in order, so I was invited to meet them in a hotel at Manchester airport.

I felt a little more confident at this one because the girls from Manchester looked a lot more like me and less like Italian supermodels. However, I was nervous and gave poor, stilted responses to questions, sadly I was not asked to wait for a second interview.

Imagine my surprise when British Caledonian put an advert in the Manchester Evening news two days later. They were having Open Interviews the following Sunday (meaning that anyone could present themselves for interview without invitation), so I put on the same dress and went along. I had a great first interview and I actually made the staff laugh at my replies, I was joyful to be asked to wait for a second interview. I entered the room for this next event and sat down, but in the back of my mind was hope that I wasn't recognised from seven days earlier.

Thankfully, none of my interviewers looked familiar at all. I relaxed again and we were in the middle of a great conversation around why I had gone to live just outside of Paris and work in a racing stable for six months aged only 18 (speaking a foreign language was a qualification) when the male interviewer looked again at my application and said these words.

"We had an applicant from your hometown last week, she worked in the same hotel as you, do you know her??? "

I was floored, what to say? Confess and risk my application being ripped up in front of me? Be rejected because I had already been found wanting once and nothing had changed for me in a week. How would they take it if I confessed that I had returned for a second attempt, perhaps they would approve of my persistence? There was a pause long enough to park a jumbo jet, then I said as calmly as I could, 'no, I don't know who that could be'. Long story short, I was offered a position three days later and cried happy tears of joy, I was joining an elite group of flight attendants and would fly the world in style.

Funnily enough, when I called hometown and spoke to an old work friend, she told me that one of our other hotel colleagues had attended that same first interview in Manchester and been accepted! We would be in training together. What were the chances of that?

Being resilient means that you can stay in a beautiful emotional state every day no matter what life throws at you, by maintaining balance between hope and despair, falling and rising, and negative self-chatter vs positive thoughts and actions. Resilience will help you to stop playing the same mental recording of hopeless despair, terror or shame and take control over your thoughts.

Grit, courage and resilience were needed in buckets when my husband very publicly flaunted his latest girlfriend under my nose, and our divorce arrived soon afterwards. All of you who are going through some stage of menopause will understand how, when hormones go haywire, relationships can suffer.

Since then my life has been wildly varied and has held extremes of wealth which has conditioned my resilience but has created a need for certainty and safety. I'm still working on those things.

"It's impossible to emerge as a goddess unless you've spent some part of your life learning how to become one "Nicole Barber-Lane – actor

Live your dreams - If you've always wanted to be a vet and found yourself in a different occupation for most of your life, you might think it's too late. I know someone who had this dream and her excuse for not following up on it was that she would be 50 by the time she qualified. I told her that she would be 50 anyway, so she should be a 50-year-old who made her dream come true. As someone who went through an arduous two-year training to become a pharmaceutical sales rep at age 47, I know how daunting it is.

These days it's perfectly possible to study and qualify in most professions from your own home. In 2016 I decided to become a certified Life Coach, something I felt 'called' to do. The course was home study, and over 9 months I discovered I was capable of so much more than I had ever imagined. Now I specialise in supporting women to keep their business, family or career flourishing through the menopause. You can discover more about my work in this area at www.freddycarrick.com

Here's a little warning. You might find that your usual circle of friends is a bit negative about you wanting to do different things and bring change into your life. This most often happens when one person meets a new romantic partner, or divorces; or loses weight.

We all need our friends to be our greatest supporters, cheering us on from the side lines of our lives. Everyone becomes like the 5 people they spend most time with, adopting and adapting to the ways and opinions of that group. We do it because we need to fit in and be a part of a tribe. This is another thing our Neanderthal brain does; it's a survival technique which means that we will never be cast out and have to fend for ourselves.

However, as Jonathon Livingston Seagull discovered, fitting in with a group that no longer fits us is really uncomfortable. Long term, trying to stay the same in order to be accepted when our soul needs to grow and change can lead to serious illness, mental and physical. Many breakdowns are really painful emotional breakthroughs when a soul resorts to drastic measures in order to achieve change.

Occasionally a woman will break the trust of others in order to join in with conversations around the water cooler or in the staff room. That little nugget of information or complaint is honey to the gossips, but a goddess would never do that because it weakens her spirit. Keep your family stories to yourself and chat about non personal stuff if you get tempted.

Adaptability – there's nothing more ageing than feeling that you are out of touch, out of date or irrelevant. Paradoxically, there's nothing more attractive than a woman who makes time every day to laugh and play and find joy in simple things. Go and play, find a new group of friends who share your hobby. Take up a new hobby, maybe something you wanted to do for years but didn't have the time because of children or parents.

I found a salsa dance class and joined it alone. Yes, I was a wee bit shy, but everyone was so welcoming that going the second time was easy. In dance classes all the ladies dance with all the men at some point, so it can be a perfect way to meet new people. Most dance classes have regular social events as well, so it isn't all about lessons.

Stay curious, be interested instead of interesting. The person who likes you most will be the person who feels that you are interested in them, not just downloading all your own stuff into the conversation. When you meet someone new, take a few minutes to find out more about them. It's true that many of the most interesting people are shy of putting themselves forward, and yet social media is full of opinions and comments from young people who have barely experienced life yet.

Self-care involves being kind and loving to yourself which will mean that you can give and be your best to those you love. It means saying no to things because you value your time. This is the time when you're allowed to say 'hell no' without instant change of mind. Being kind to yourself means putting an end to the endless 'what if' mind chatter and the 'I should have' stuff that makes you squirm as you remember. Stop it.

Learning how to appreciate your life as it is and not how you think it should be is the secret to peace in your heart. That, along with not being tempted to make your problems or situation any worse than it actually is in order to feed your 'worry bear'.

Self-knowledge is a gift that only time, and experience will bring. Luxuriate in it.

Find a purpose – something which excites you; think of something you would like to be involved in or you would like to set up to serve a section of community, or a whole community. If you have spare time, then make it matter. If you're content and fulfilled by baking cakes for others and tending your garden, do that. Just make sure that whatever you do in your spare time is something that makes you happy and brings a smile of anticipation when you think about it. According to Globalentrepreneurship.com, over the last decade the highest rate of business start-up activity globally is in the over 55s. If you have a bit of available pension to spend you could do worse than invest it in yourself. There's so much choice of what you could do; personal development courses, new skills training, buying some leisure time by paying someone else to clean your home or do your ironing. Perhaps you might re-design your garden to make it less time-consuming or start a small business.

Another statistic to note is that by 2024 over 25% of workers will be females over 55. That is a lot of women who will need to be catered for in the workplace, meaning there's plenty of opportunity to begin small businesses for that demographic. It might be a side hustle such as selling skin care and personal items for busy working women who have no time for that type of shopping. It might be providing personal assistant type support or teaching your skills online to a thousand raving fans.

Everyone just wants to feel happy, that's all, just happy

Leadership – I knew I was a leader when I was 8 years old and along the way I forgot, allowing myself to be consumed by doubts and fears; now I'm at the other end of life, I know that leadership begins with what is in my heart, not my thoughts. The beauty and love I feel for all, the compassion and support, spreads through my team and can spread through a room and a company.

I behave with leadership; I mean that I am prepared to lead others where they want to go. That may be towards better health, as within my fitness business; education in particular areas, this book for example, and subsequent workshops. or guiding people in personal development to discover the life they imagined when they were children. I do this through my group and individual coaching sessions.

A goddess is often a leader simply because she has high standards and others will want to be around her. You can lead others to do anything so long as your leadership comes from your heart and is for the greater good. Anyone who attempts to lead because they like the power or prestige of being in charge is less likely to succeed long-term unless they stoop to fear, manipulation or bullying tactics.

Now my business is something I dreamed of. For many years I was a tiny cog in a large corporate machine, and these days I love knowing that every day something new will develop. Whether it's an idea for a blog post or a podcast, or the beginnings of a new book, a meeting with collaborators – every new idea is an opportunity to support other women in their search for freedom, whatever they hope to be free from.

Presence – is the ability to focus on what is happening around you to the elimination of distractions. When you have a conversation with someone, it's very normal to listen with one ear and have your brain thinking of what you're going to say next. The other person will know what you're doing, however, because your eyes tell them. If you don't believe me, go and have a chat with someone who is likely to respond to everything you say with either their own view on your situation, or their own much worse story on the same subject. Pay attention to their body language and eyes, you can feel if they're listening to listen or listening to speak.

Being present in a conversation would mean that you listen with both ears and stay focussed until the other stops speaking. Then, give yourself a few heartbeats to consider your response. This is hugely effective in every single conversation you have with everyone you meet. Your children or partner will feel seen and heard by you when you behave with presence.

You are truly unique; only you have the experiences and skills gathered over your lifetime. You may think that you're of no consequence, but to many younger women, your wisdom is what they need. You might feel you've achieved little over the years, but I urge you to sit down and write your own biography. It doesn't have to be detailed or elaborate, just write and acknowledge the things you have achieved, then have a little celebration either with yourself or a trusted friend.

Teach others some of the things you know, even if they are in competition. I see this on YouTube and Facebook all the time. There's an infinite abundance in this world with plenty for everyone, therefore there's no longer any need to be secretive or mean with your skills.

Charisma – as well as demonstrating leadership, a goddess is charismatic; these types of people are generally optimistic and have a pleasant and cheerful attitude. Others like to be around them because they will usually try to see the best in everyone.

A woman who has a sincere smile and is good at maintaining eye contact, can be really good at influencing others. When people know they are being treated fairly and well, and are enthused by someone to do better, they will usually try to achieve their best.

One thing you can do which is certain to be for the greater good is to learn more about menopause and set up self-help groups in your workplace or community. Make sure that the next generation of younger women, and the one after that, know what to expect and when. They will then feel safe discussing it in their workplace because it will be as much a part of the conversation as last night's TV or the weather. When you are ready to do this, you'll find more information and support on the ACAS website.

Confidence – I am not perfect, in actual fact, I am regularly a wee bit broken; happily, I've learnt that I can fix myself fairly quickly.

By the time I was 45 I finally understood that my energy and confidence go through cycles; the major ones last 7 or 14 years, but there are minor ones too, lasting a few days. Being aware of the cycles and understanding them helps me because I know that If I'm having an 'off' day, tomorrow will probably be better. If tomorrow is no better, I absolutely know that the next day will be, because my low mood never lasts more than 2 days. Unless I allow it to. I've learnt some tricks for getting out of a poor state; taught by the best mindset trainers in the World.

So, once I notice I'm feeling low and not reacting well to whatever is going on around me, I need to use those tricks. To switch from being in a poor state to a happy and creative one, where energy is increased and I can look outside of myself with a positive and happier attitude, I take these steps.

1. I listen to loud music and dance; it's not possible to feel dreadful when I'm jigging around my kitchen or bouncing on my rebounder to Springsteen screaming No Surrender. This is called **changing my physical state** and it's important because it can be too easy to stay in a slump, feeling negative.

   If you are at work, you can change your state by finding a staircase and running up a few flights, and down as you're smiling or laughing. You could walk briskly around some part of the building for 2/3 minutes, find a place where you can do some squats or a little bit of jogging on the spot.

   At home, you can dance yourself out of misery or go and have a lovely bath or shower. Last year I learnt a trick which I never would have believed I would use regularly. I began to turn my shower onto its coldest setting at the end and stand in it for as long as I could. I can do 90 seconds but longer would be better.

   The trick for success is to breath and relax and hold onto something because I usually end up giggling and squealing. Doctors have discovered that this will encourage your lymph glands to clean themselves out. Efficient lymph glands keep your body healthy and help to reduce inflammation which causes cancer, heart disease and arthritis. The payoff is that I come out of my shower smiling and that joy stays with me for hours; a silly, childish, gleeful amount of joy.

   Think about it and decide on something you can do to alter your physical state whenever you feel lethargic, stuck, despondent or depressed.

2. I maintain a level of structure around the various projects I have going on at any time. Small projects such as planting bulbs for the next season, or bigger projects such as building my business or planning my next foreign trip. A lot of focus goes into these projects,
   and whether you write your plans down or not, I know you make them too, because we all have to plan forward. It doesn't matter if it's organising a birthday party, packing for a weekend visit to friends, or going on a shopping trip with a friend.

These plans are where my focus should be but I'm human, and my focus very regularly shifts to dark places. The dark places seem to appear whenever I feel stressed, tired or under pressure to do something I really don't feel comfortable about; then my old patterns of behaviour can assert themselves and I can drift down into a feeling of hopelessness and inadequacy really quickly.

That small negative voice of fear reminds me that I can't achieve this plan because of (things from the past), or thinking that's a useless idea (who do I think I am to try and do that?) then sometimes, it's too tempting to listen to that voice and abandon the plan.

As soon as I notice this has happened and I'm daydreaming my way into oblivion, I need to do something to **change my focus.** The well-known phrase "where focus goes, energy flows" is true, so I've learnt to acknowledge the voice of fear, soothe it with kind words, but tell it firmly that I'm not a little girl anymore and I can do this. Then I can put attention back into my plan and take the next step towards making things happen.

Being resilient means that you can stay in a beautiful emotional state every day no matter what life throws at you, by maintaining balance between hope and despair, falling and rising, and negative self-chatter vs positive thoughts and actions. Resilience will help you to stop playing the same mental recording of hopeless despair, terror or shame, and take control over your thoughts.

3. I've learnt that the language I use to myself and others creates the way I feel; alternately, the way I feel is because of the language I use to describe a situation. I learnt to **change my language** and my belief about my story.

In the past I used to say that I'm not a person who 'does detail', but these days I acknowledge that I'm an 'ideas' person and I hire others to finish the details.

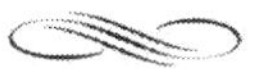

We all have stories about our lives and the events that have shaped us. We learn them as children and by the time we're adults, the stories are actually our history. Most of us go around telling the same stories to every new person we meet, thus positioning ourselves as a victim, hero, peacemaker, achiever, or whatever.

Humans have a tendency re-live events and conversations which happened decades ago, word perfect in our own minds. Finally understanding that the past is not my future unless I continue to live in it, was a game changer for me. I had to find a way to change those old stories and stop punishing myself for my past mistakes. Soiling my future by constantly reminding myself of my past is unhealthy and unhelpful. I had to forgive myself, grow from what I learnt, and move on with life.

In his books titled the Curious Brain Hack to Build Inner Strength, and Hardwire Happiness, Dr Rick Hanson PhD, suggests that we have the power to use our minds to change our brains which can change our minds for the better. I was comforted to realise I could change all the old limiting stories I'd been telling myself for years. Stories I told others to explain the way I behave and the things I do, or don't do.

Dr Hanson has an idea that we have three parts of the mind which he has named a mouse, a lizard and a monkey. Each of the three need to be nourished each day in order to create a holistic sense of connectedness and belonging within ourselves. Being kind to ourselves and looking for opportunities to register feelings of happiness and gratitude every day, are useful to build inner resilience.

Within all of us is a prime need to feel safe and reassured, so if you regularly feel defensive, misunderstood or stressed, you might need to make some radical changes in your work or home life. No matter the sadness you face in your life or the challenges, you can change your future by realising that everyday there are opportunities to experience something good.

Be happy for others, that's a complete antidote to disappointment and envy – just say, that's great, I'm happy for you and mean it for a second or two. You'll feel better. Being envious or resentful is like drinking poison and waiting for the other person to die.

When you deflect a compliment because you feel that by accepting it you are being conceited, then you are rejecting a loving comment, and therefore the love of the person giving you the compliment.

Years ago, I attended a workshop on personal healing and one practice I learnt there has stayed with me ever since. It's the ability to accept a compliment with grace. It sounds like a very simple practice, but it isn't because a woman's reflex is to disagree with the person paying the compliment. This totally negates her opportunities to hold onto lovely moments which can be turned into positive pathways in her brain, I bet you know someone who does this, or maybe you do too.

My question to you is, does your old story still fit you? I mean, if you're reading this book you will probably be older than 35; perhaps it's time for a new story, or at least a new chapter. One that's fitting for a magnificent woman living the best years of her life with grace and vitality.

Of course, it might be a bit tricky to expect your family and old friends or long-term work colleagues to hear your new story, but you don't have to tell it to them straight away. You just need to tell it to yourself, often, while you smile into the mirror, and while you walk your dog or walk around the grocery store.

When you're ready to tell this new story to people who know you well, here's an idea. My new stories begin with "in the past I... but these days I..." those words will tell my voice of fear that I no longer believe my old stories and am ready to use my new story. Try it, think about a self-belief which is negative, and change it.

Goddess = wisdom, understanding, compassion, intuition, balance

In his book The Mind Body Connection, Deepak Chopra demonstrates how every cell in our body is listening to our emotional thoughts and reacts accordingly. Deepak tells us that every emotional state has a chemical counterpart in the brain called a neuropeptide. Those chemicals send messages to every cell in the body to behave in certain ways. Therefore, if you constantly tell yourself that you're too old, or useless, or a poor something, then your body will believe you and behave accordingly.

If you tell yourself daily that you are brilliant, beautiful and bright, then your body will believe you.

Neuroplasticity - is a relatively new science which understands that it is possible to rewire your brain using only thoughts. This is what Deepak Chopra and Rick Hanson are talking about. It's now known that everything you think creates feelings, and those feelings create behaviours. Repeated behaviours create habits within your speech, relationships, work, environment, in fact everything which influences your biology, and therefore, your brain. This is why positive self-talk works so well and regular use of personal 'incantations' so effective.

Think of some things you can say to yourself every day to make you feel fantastic and powerful and successful in everything you attempt. Begin each one with 'I am...' because that is how you tell your brain what you want it to react to. Here are some I use:

- I am healthy, I am wealthy, I am generous, I am kind; I am 100% in my body and mind
- I am joyful and playful, I am thankful for laughter
- I am dynamic, brilliant and bright, I'm a radiant being of light
- I am an expert in female menopause
- I am a generous, loving and dependable friend
- I am a fountain of wealth; love, health and money flow through me with ease

when you stop growing you start dying, like a flower

Neurobics – is the science of brain exercise. Its primary goal is to help maintain your memory, as well as honing your ability to learn new information. The term neurobics was coined by Lawrence Katz, Ph.D. and Manning Rubin to describe such brain exercises; it includes many practices that help the brain to stay fit and young.

Those brain exercises are activities that stimulate the brain, prevent memory loss and improve memory recall. Just like physical exercise which creates greater, stronger muscle tissue, neurobics will stimulate the brain to increase its neural pathways and make them work harder.

Neurobics =mental exercises create new brain pathways, which create a bigger hippocampus = better memory and stronger brain power

You've heard the phrase 'use it or lose it'; in this context it means that you need to challenge your brain every day to stimulate the far corners of it. Clearly you don't want to have your brain working at 100% all day because that would be exhausting. Asking your brain for more effort occasionally through the day though, is helpful and healthy.

Neural activity is stimulated by asking the brain to perform habitual tasks in a different way. For example; writing with your non-dominant hand every day for short periods of time, learning a new language, even beginning to walk using the other leg to the one you usually stride out on. Simple things like lifting the non-dominant foot to go first when you walk upstairs and cleaning your teeth with the 'other' hand, will make your brain and whole body re-think its usual habits.

None of these suggestions need to be taken to extremes to be effective. You don't need to be a fluent speaker of Arabic, a grade 5 saxophone player, or to be writing letters with your 'other' hand. In these exercises you are asking your brain to tell your body to behave differently to the way it behaves out of habit. This difference will increase the blood flow in your brain which increases the production of happiness chemicals and will create a feeling of joy and fulfilment.

Another benefit is a feeling of satisfaction that you have challenged yourself and succeeded, which is a great reason to congratulate yourself on achieving something new.

BNDF (brain derived neurotrophic factor) is a protein that grows nerve cells linked to brain power, it is boosted with wrong hand activity – and doing something new

Worry – is really the most useless emotion we can 'do' because it absolutely achieves nothing.

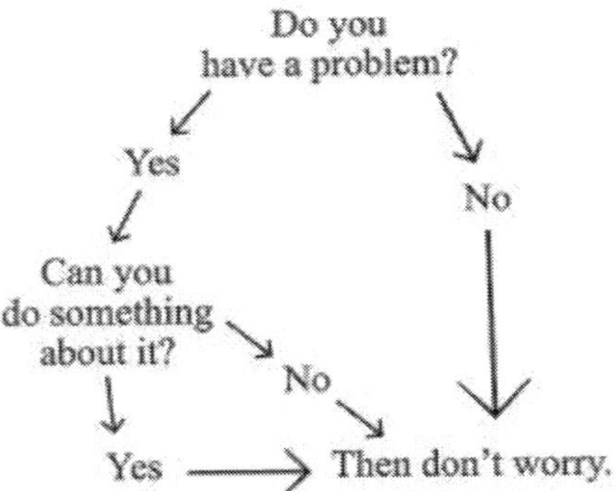

Research suggests that 40% of everything we worry about may never happen, 30% has already happened and we can do nothing to change the outcome, and 12% are needless worries where we create possible outcomes and then fret about them

There is a difference between worry and anxiety; nearly every person alive indulges in worrying about potential or past events, while it's far less common for people to develop anxiety over potential or past events. The main difference is that the two states affect your body in different ways.

If the solution you came up with is to take action over the worry and you don't, you're likely to continue to worry about the same situation regularly. The saying 'a coward dies a thousand deaths, but a brave person dies only once' means that a coward will decide on action to take and never take it, thus continuing to worry and ultimately feeling personal disappointment over lack of action. A brave woman will decide on action and then take it, she will say what needs to be said, remove whatever needs to be removed from her life or even decide not to do the thing that has caused the worry; but she moves on, having made a decision.

Worry can cause a temporary change of emotional state, but anxiety lasts longer. Usually, once we find a solution the feeling of worry can go away, but when you're anxious about life, the focus of this anxiety can switch from one situation to another, causing you to feel stressed all the time.

Worry tends to be more of a 'loop' of thoughts around a particular situation or problem, and sometimes this actually creates solutions to the cause of worry. Whereas feelings of anxiety can be transferred onto anything else which a person isn't certain about.

We are the only animal species on earth which can think a thought and become afraid or angry or worried or embarrassed. So, our minds can actually create a stress situation, even though we might just be lying in bed waiting for sleep. Cortisol is always produced when your mind thinks about stress situations and you allow your body to go into its 'fight or flight' reaction. You'll recognise that state because you will notice that your breath is shallow and faster, and your heart rate speeds up.

If you feel you suffer from anxiety and it stops you living your life the way you want to, then some cognitive behaviour therapy or personal coaching could be the answer. If your anxiety is really holding you back in life then talking to your doctor might help and, if it's appropriate, a course of medication.

While going through my periods of depression, my therapist suggested that I gave myself a time every day when it was ok and safe to 'do worry'. There is good research to prove that by giving yourself permission to worry, it isn't quite such a big deal. Also, if you find yourself 'doing worry' outside of the allotted time slot, you could take control and tell yourself that this worry can wait until later. Studies have shown that those who scheduled time to worry experienced a significant decrease in anxiety compared to those in the study who worried randomly throughout the day.

Goddess – a woman adored

Feminine appearance - I attended a personal development event last year which took place over six long days, working well into the night. I began the week in leggings and sweatshirt but on the fourth day I wore a dress and leggings; the fifth day I tied a silk scarf around my neck with a bow. It was a real surprise to me how different I felt with those small tweaks to my appearance, but more important, was the difference in how others reacted towards me. Those small touches of femininity caused me to move and behave more like a woman, and I loved it.

Being seen requires you to show yourself in your glorious authenticity. If it's wearing gym gear all day and bouncing along in trainers do that. If it's with voluminous clothing and spiky silver hair then that's what it is, but you know what – it's your smile and the way you hold yourself that people notice.

My hair has evolved over the last few years from long and coloured blond to short and silver. I decided to begin highlighting my long hair once the hair parting glimmered white, and the frequent full head colour was a chore. The result was that my silver hair mingled with the blond highlights which I liked, and it stayed that way for a few years. Over time, I had fewer blond highlights applied and longer between re-touching. Finally, I just allowed the highlights to fade and stopped re-touching altogether.

Silver is having a trend at present and Jane Fonda has decided to be an influencer. Her silver hair made its debut at the Oscars this year and Sharon Osbourne quickly followed suit; I'm wondering who will be next and hoping that it's Joanna Lumley.

A lot of women compliment my hair colour with a comment that their hair is very salt and pepper, or not a very attractive grey. I tell them that it will get lighter with time but choosing to continue to colour their hair is personal. I can point you to a Facebook group called GGG or @GoingGrayGuide, where you'll find a ton of fabulous women either totally or partially grey. One thing that is noticeable from all the photos posted on that group is all the women look more relaxed in their authentic grey and their complexions look so much softer and younger.

Family - develop some kind of code within your home so that your family know why you're irrational or tearful or totally unreasonable, just because they asked for clean socks.

When a parent is out of balance, feeling irritable and grumpy it's harder to feel benevolent towards the family. A woman in perimenopause may have school aged children who need a level of consistency and structure. Brain fog and poor concentration often means that meetings and events at school might be forgotten, and this lack of efficiency can show up at work too.

A modern goddess is strong, balanced and 'cool'. She keeps a careful eye on the health of her family but especially on her own. What's the point of having a fantastic trampoline in the garden if you're too unfit to get onto it, let alone bounce around on it?

If your children are old enough, and you are able to sit your family down for an open discussion about how you are feeling and why you're not behaving the way they are used to, then it really is a good idea to do that. To involve your family in something that affects all of them and ask for their support and help is a sign of a good leader.

Teenagers may be reluctant to hear you but giving them some responsibility is a good thing. As I mentioned earlier, your behaviour during menopause may have some comparison to the behaviour of your teenage children. I mean that hormonal fluctuations cause the same emotional upheaval, irrespective of the age when they happen. Perhaps sometimes you could make the family laugh by reminding them that if they notice you behaving in a stroppy and irrational way it's likely to be menopause.

Your partner needs another conversation however, and this one needs some level of open discussion around sexual challenges as well as extra emotional support which will give you a huge boost (see the chapter on Menopause Vagina). If your partner doesn't know what's happening with you and how much help you need, how can your fluctuating moods and faded libido be understood? It might be the only period of time that you've been vulnerable within the relationship, but there's extra intimacy and trust which can build from that.

Your family need some idea of how long this will continue, you can honestly tell them you don't know, but probably around five years or maybe ten!

Posture – the way you move tells people so much more about your physical and mental health, your confidence, and your age than facial wrinkles ever will. I recently took a walk with a friend and had to comment on the way she moved, it was so feminine in a way I could see but not describe. Taking meaningful exercise regularly and doing everything you can to stay supple will keep you moving easily and will maintain a degree of tone in your muscles, and therefore your skin.

When I taught aerobics, I would tell the class that every session was a building block on the path to long term health. I still have great stamina and strong bones; I don't have flabby arms and my thighs are strong; I hope many of my clients are still in good shape too.

- When you walk a little taller and straighter, there are many hidden but important things going on inside of you:
- Shoulders are down and further back, giving your neck muscles a rest
- It's easier to smile because your face is more relaxed
- Your back is straighter which, over time will subtly shift the whole way you walk
- Your hips will take less strain because your back is straighter
- Your knees will move more freely because your hips are relaxed
- Your digestive system improves because you're standing straighter and taller

These benefits could happen just because you painted your toenails. If you like the feeling, then you may want to change other things in your life as well. For example, once you feel the benefits of better posture through your neck and spine, it could be a great idea to take more and longer walks or sign up for a stretch class or beginners' yoga.

It's only a short step now to making some changes in your diet which will bring more feelings of dopamine and serotonin release because clothes will fit better and, over a short period of time, you will feel brighter mentally as well as have more energy. Being slim, fit and healthy is a strong preference for me so I will do whatever it takes to stay that way.

Health - bearing in mind every cell in my body will be different in 5 years' time, I can repair, like magic. If something is wrong, I can fix it as long as my cells are healthy, and the problem isn't terminal. I recently met and got to know two young men who are limbless and absolutely crushing it on the public speaker platform.

As I told you in the chapter around weight gain, I re-modelled my physical self a couple of years ago and, although I have been known to enjoy a substantial helping of pudding and/or chocolates at times, I do still make my green blend on at least three days every week.

The idea of starvation never appealed to me, but that feeling of being light instead of full and of being energetic instead of lethargic, makes every bag of spinach worthwhile. Most days I don't eat anything between my evening meal and breakfast, except water and a hot drink before bed. This is a small nod towards daily fasting, it keeps my bowels working well and my stomach flatter.

Every writer of books based on healthy eating will encourage you to allow your body to completely digest what you eat, and rest after eating it. If your tummy is bloated, imagine all the food you ate over several days literally 'backed up' in your digestive system. A bit like the M3 at Dover when the English Channel is too rough for ferries to sail. Just think of a lorry loaded with bread being pushed along by another lorry full of vegetables, then pasta and sauce and putrid meat compacted by chocolate and doughnuts and crisps and more bread and fermenting fruit – is it any wonder that the gas we pass smells!

I've said already that I'm not a nutritionist, but many women declare that changing their diet has helped to relieve some of their menopause symptoms.

when you give up the hope of staying fit and active, then old age runs to meet you

Having written all of the above I want you to know that, should you find yourself sitting alone in your garden because you've had an argument with loved ones, and you're entertaining thoughts that the family will be better off without you, you need to sing the last few lines of 'I AM WOMAN' by Helen Reddy and then ask for support from people who understand what's happening to you. Talk to your doctor or practice nurse, a friend or colleague who might have been through your stage of life already. Just ask for support because it's always available.

WHO STOLE MY WOMAN?

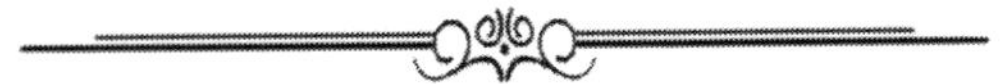

5 things men need to understand about menopause, plus some more stuff

Hi, have you noticed a few things are different in your relationship recently?

A woman I know was so distressed over her own behaviour that she left her husband and young teenage son and moved back in with her parents. Having no idea whatsoever what was happening to her and unable to manage her mood swings, she decided that her family would be better off without her.

Her lovely husband persuaded her to talk to a menopause specialist who helped her understand how the menopause can affect even the most level-headed of women. She's now back with her family and managing the situation much better but will never forget how she was willing to give up everything she loved because of her lack of knowledge around the menopause.

Here are a few reasons why you might not know what your lady is going through at present: -

- First of all, she isn't going mad, in spite of changing behaviours
- It could be that she doesn't know herself and is confused

- She might be frightened that she's out of control occasionally and doesn't know what to do about it
- Have you noticed she's a bit forgetful recently? I bet she has
- Does she turn away from you when you go to give a cuddle or a kiss?
- Do you worry she's having an affair?
- Does she keep you awake with her tossing and turning through the night, up and down to the bathroom and needing to change her nightwear or bedsheets more than she used to?
- Has she asked you to read this or left it open where you'll pick it up?

Another woman I know is very senior in her career and mother of grown children. She felt so unstable that she disappeared from home one day and drove hundreds of miles, stopping only when she arrived at the home of her grandmother. Her husband was frantic because she took only her handbag with her and gave him no hint of anything wrong. Police were called and traced her by her car registration. Thankfully, she is also now back home with all the support of her lovely husband and is now taking HRT.

Been with husband 19 years but just can't get on now. He doesn't understand what we go through and just blames everything on me and the menopause. Haven't slept in same room for about 5 years anyway cause of my night sweats and his snoring. He is so rude and nasty to me and I wonder if that is affecting me as much as the menopause is.

In brief: -

The menopause happens to every woman who has gone through puberty and it's actually very much like puberty, but in reverse. I mean; instead of her hormone factory *beginning* to produce female reproductive hormones, it is *closing down* production of those hormones. The resulting mood swings and volcanic fury is pretty similar, but more devastating because now she has to take responsibility for many areas of her life, whereas in puberty, responsibility was left to parents. It's a hormonal transition often also called 'the change'. Firstly, due to lack of education around the subject, she isn't expecting to be menopausal until early 50s. When she's 50, she expects she might notice a few hot flushes occasionally over a couple of years, and then it'll be over. Until this last year, no-one has educated women to expect anything else. However, as the hormone factory slows down production, the shortage of hormones slowly but surely becomes a problem.

The years during which the factory is slowly closing down is called perimenopause, (the time before menopause) and can last between 4 and 8 years.

This is the moment to say that no two women will have the same experience, so just because your Mum or your sister went through perimenopause and menopause with no problems, doesn't mean your own partner will. Around 75% of women do have symptoms bad enough to significantly reduce their (and their family's) quality of life.

The average age of a woman reaching total menopause is 51, so early to middle forties is when a woman might expect to notice her first symptoms. Once over 51, she is no longer fertile, the ovaries have finished their redundancy consultation period and her monthly bleeds have stopped for at least 12 months; now she's medically described as postmenopausal. This period of time after the age of 51 is when the earlier symptoms continue, and some new ones come into play.

A woman produces three hormones which affect reproduction; these are oestrogen, progesterone and testosterone. Women produce around twice as much testosterone as oestrogen over their lifetime. During the 'redundancy consultation period' the production of progesterone and oestrogen becomes erratic and eventually stops. Testosterone takes a little longer to stop and that can be why many women in menopause transition become 'thicker' around the middle, taking a more masculine shape.

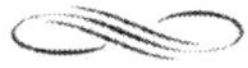

AS HER LOVING PARTNER, YOU NEED TO KNOW

Signs/symptoms of the perimenopause

If your partner isn't using any hormonal contraception, the first sign will probably be that her monthly bleeding is disrupted, a nasty effect because women really like to know when to be ready for that. Men have no clue how disruptive and embarrassing it can be for a woman to be caught without any sanitary products in her bag. If taking hormonal contraception, this symptom will be greatly reduced or non-existent during the perimenopause stage.

The next obvious sign is when she starts to become forgetful or disorganised, you might notice a lack of focus or concentration. Women complain of bursting into tears for no reason, and generally feeling unhappy and sad. For many women, this can go unnoticed for years, until she begins to think she's losing her mind. In fact, many women ask their doctor for a referral to the Elderly Care Consultant because they worry that they're slipping into dementia.

An obvious link to that sign is that she may become unreasonably angry and irrational over the smallest challenge or mistake. It can be breath-taking how fast a woman can go from lovely to lunatic and you may feel there's nothing you can do to help her feel better; there is, and I'll tell you later what it is. The level of oestrogen produced by her body is changing almost daily, so it's not surprising that her moods fluctuate.

Sleeping problems will affect both of you if you share a bed; the sign of perimenopause that no woman can escape is the wild temperature control. Hot flushes and night sweats are the very devils work and if neither of you sleeps well for weeks or months it will become a major problem. You could try using single duvets on your large bed, just as the Europeans do, and see if that helps. Keeping the bedroom cool and a window open also can help. Research shows that having a duvet filled with wool instead of synthetic padding or feathers, is very helpful.

Many women lose confidence in themselves and their abilities during these years and can become anxious about things they used to manage very well before. 12% of women decide they want to retire from work or reduce their working hours during this time, simply because of their anxiety, mood swings, weariness and forgetfulness.

There are other, less specific signs and symptoms of the perimenopause, such as she may complain she aches all the time, and hips are a real problem in early morning.

Muscles ache and she might be feeling tired all the time. If she's lacking in energy, confidence and generally lethargic about keeping up with exercise or social events, YOUR life will be different. Many women lose weight during these years, but just as many put weight on, especially around the midriff. It can look really 'middle aged' and speaking for myself, I hated that my midriff spread down to my stomach area and didn't seem to end until my thighs.

Let's talk about sex and the lost libido.

The most confusing symptom of all for a woman is why she no longer wants to be intimate with a partner she's had years of loving with. I think it's unlikely that she will start a conversation around this and if you feel that each time you go for a cuddle or just to kiss her, she turns away, then you could be forgiven for taking it personally.

Many men I speak to talk about the emotional isolation and sadness they feel that their emotional connection has broken down. Let me explain a little about what might be going on.

We all know how fickle a thing 'desire' is and how it fluctuates without reason. When her oestrogen is low, it can cause a woman to feel undesirable, as well as reducing her sex drive. Please note that when she feels undesirable, she won't be making any moves towards you, at all, ever.

Also, there are changes inside of her vagina which are caused by the lower levels of oestrogen, these changes are a major cause of the reduction in your sex life.

When the supply of oestrogen changes, the balance of acid and alkaline in some parts of the body changes too. The result of that can cause the 'good bacteria' (which keeps certain areas healthy) to go out of balance as well, and that's most noticeable when more 'gas' is produced. This change in bacteria may also create problems around the bladder and vagina. The result is that urinary infection is common, and there can be a discoloured discharge which sometimes has a kind of 'fishy' odour. Some women are so embarrassed by this particular symptom they take themselves off to the sexual health department in the hospital, thinking they have developed something nasty.

Most importantly, the change in levels of oestrogen can cause the skin around the bladder and vagina to be drier and thinner. The result of that is she will possibly need to pee a lot more often and having intercourse can be like sticking a knife into her. She might feel that her internal skin is tearing and be afraid of damage. Again, this isn't a symptom that women discuss between themselves, so it's unlikely that she will tell you. I hope you can understand how all of these developments can make her afraid to let you close. Sadly, using more lubricant isn't an especially helpful answer, but vaginal moisturisers are available and can make a difference. However, if you do use lube, make sure it's non-perfumed, is paraben and glycerine free, and is pH balanced.

This is a comment from a friend *"I'm only 46 and everything went downhill last year – hated the periods being all over the shop, hot flushes, tired, no sex drive, boobs massive, you name it I had it. My mum was earlier with perimenopause, so I just thought I'm not suffering anymore. But HRT is great, honestly feel so much better – moods improved, sex drive getting there, vaginal dryness gone "*

It's obvious that this lack of physical intimacy, over a period of time, could lead to either or both parties feeling frustrated and isolated in their confusion. It doesn't need to be that way though, because now that you both have a better understanding of 'why' your lives have changed, then you can talk it through and plan a better future.

The menopause can be a time of great freedom for women, so it's worth a celebration of some wonderful years to come.

So, what could go wrong?

You can help by getting educated and being supportive

Remember, it's not about you.

When women reach their late forties and fifties they begin to feel not seen, overlooked, not heard, disregarded. No wonder women lose confidence in their abilities. If you really pay attention to this woman, so that you can see her properly and not just the outline of someone you spend a lot of time with, then you will notice when her behaviour changes. The behaviours described above are behaviours that she has little control over, she's not going mad but is probably feeling constantly guilty over her anger, her forgetfulness and her inability to talk to you.

Another comment from a friend "*Decided we would split up today. Don't even feel like I care about him and am fed up of the arguments and him shouting at me. Sorry think I just needed to write this. Am sat here not knowing what to do right now. Also, I've been on antidepressants for about 5 years for menopause*"

However, now that you know a bit more, you might persuade her to go and have a chat with her doctor and go with her if she agrees. Do some research yourself on what kind of remedies are available, and what hormone therapy is all about. Women regularly complain that the doctor doesn't know enough about menopause to help, so take along the N.I.C.E. guidance to show him. You can find this guidance on a website called @NewsonHealth, so can your doctor.

The reason she might resist this is because if you mention the word 'menopause' she's likely to get more upset. Accepting that she might be menopausal is accepting the end of her fertility and she thinks she is now OLD, and every woman really wants to feel they're OLD, don't they?

Her colleagues might already have given up on her as a person who is punctual and reliable and, in the UK, 12% of women decide to give up their career because they lose confidence and feel incapable.

There, there, it'll be alright

There are frequent stories of men who 'trade in their middle-aged wives for younger models'. Two reasons why it isn't such a smart move and one why it might be.

- Every woman beyond puberty will go through the menopause at some time
- Your long-term partner has shared many years of history with you that no-one else knows

- Your younger partner MIGHT be willing to be your nurse in a few years

What your long-term partner fears above most other things, is being left for a younger woman. In exactly the same way that you would be afraid of being left if you develop erectile dysfunction, which is more and more common.

There is something that you can do with her every single day to make sure she continues to feel safe and loved and valued in your partnership. Now you know what's happening and understand how it affects every aspect of your lives together, you have no excuses not to do this.

Warning: if she has been avoiding sex or intimate contact for a while, she may reject you at first, but persevere because this one thing will change your lives.

Gentlemen, your woman needs to be held in a safe embrace which has no sexual tone whatsoever. If you do this regularly and she learns that you're not just cuddling because you hope to have sex, then I promise she will soon feel safe and SHE will initiate more intimate moments. As soon as she feels any sexual undertone, or your trouser snake wakes up, she'll push you away and feel angry.

Here's how it goes:

- Open your arms and invite her in
- Think about holding a child and have the same neutral thoughts
- Stand strong and allow her to relax
- Breath regularly but don't be heavy
- Hold her for as long as she wants to stay there, 10 seconds or five minutes
- Do not stroke, pat, or try to kiss her
- Do not twitch any muscle that might signal the end of the embrace
- When she moves to let go, let her go without kissing her, she may kiss you but that doesn't mean sex is next.

If you do this well enough often enough, then I promise you that intimacy will return, on her terms. Maybe not full sex, but warmer cuddling and laughter definitely. Why? Because she feels safe and understood and seen, that's why.

Don't say these things

If your partner tells you she thinks she might be menopausal, don't suggest she's not that old.

Don't say your mother, aunt, boss, went through menopause with no problems because it implies there's something wrong with your woman if she complains. Every woman is different, and many go through childbirth with no painkillers where other women need epidural pain relief or caesarean.

- Please don't tell her to go and get it sorted, not helpful.
- Don't tell her she's putting weight on, if she is, she will know.
- Don't ask her if she's still going through it after a year or so, not if you want to live another day, anyway.
- When she doesn't want to go out because she's worried about having a hot flush in front of others, try to understand and order takeaway instead.
- Don't point out that her top lip is sweaty, she will know and hate that you noticed.
- Don't tell her that your mate's wife used black cohosh and never had any more problems. It's possibly not true and she will hate that you think she hasn't done her best to find a remedy.
- Don't remind her that drinking caffeine or alcohol will give more hot flushes, or you might soon be wearing the caffeine
- When she snaps at you, take a breath and walk away; ask her what you can do to help, and she will probably say 'nothing' - THIS IS YOUR CUE TO OPEN YOUR ARMS AND HOLD HER

Finally, if you manage women in the workplace, please find out what your company can do to provide more support for women working through their perimenopause and menopause. Understand more about the challenges she may face in her working day, and let your team know that you are open to this type of conversation. I hear many women being offered a fan for their desk which is kind, but unless you offer them to every desk, you may as well hang a sign from hers saying *'step away from the menopausal lady, volcanic eruptions imminent'.*

MENOPAUSE QUIZ FOR PARTNERS

1 Question: how many days in the month is your loving partner irritable?

Answer: never, whatever is the problem with a menopausal woman - it's always your fault, fact.

2 Question: when does a female become unhinged by hormones?

1. Puberty
2. Always
3. Whenever you ask for sex

Answer: 1. females are at the mercy of hormonal fluctuations from puberty until end of life, fact.

3 Question: how many times have you emptied the dishwasher in the last month?

Answer: according to her never, because in her mind she always has to empty it

4 Question: how many years do the symptoms of menopause last?

1. 2
2. 6
3. 10 or more

Answer: every woman has her own pace, average is six to ten, but if you don't empty the dishwasher the answer will be 'for the rest of your life together'.

5 Question: which symptom of the menopause does your loving partner dislike the most?

1. Developing a 'pot belly' overnight
2. Crying for no reason
3. Hot flushes that leave her dripping in sweat
4. Peeing herself when she laughs, or coughs, or moves
5. Night-time hokey-cokey with her legs and arms in and out of bed
6. Developing a dry, smelly vagina which she thinks is a disease, or cancer
7. Not wanting sex with you because of a dry, smelly vagina

Answer: any or all of the above

6 Question: what is the primary feeling that your loving partner needs from you

1. A feeling that you listen to her and you hear her?
2. A feeling that you look at her and see her?
3. A feeling of safety within your relationship?

Answer: above all things, a woman who feels safe in a loving relationship is stronger, more open (sexually) and confident than a woman who does not. If you read the full chapter, I'm going to tell you the easiest way to help her feel safe.

ACKNOWLEDGMENTS

My mother died in 2018 and aside from the grief of her death, the trauma of volcanic familial quarrels, betrayal, and dispute left me tumbling down a dark hole with nothing to hold onto. During the following eighteen months I was sustained only by the love, patience and understanding of my remaining family, Chris, Paul and Maggie, as well as dear friend Diane. Writing this book gave me a rock to steady myself on and a distraction when the pain was too much.

I'm deeply grateful to the support, encouragement and guidance I have in constant supply from all my friends within the Tony Robbins community. When I'm in your presence I feel totally understood, accepted and beloved. It's always my intention to show up amongst you with energy and vitality to lead others along the path you've shown me.

Deepest thanks to Aurora Almadori, MBBS, MSc, PhD, who is a Plastic Surgeon with specialist interest in vulval reconstruction. She generously gave me her support as well as her own research into all things vaginal while giving birth herself. Aurora juggles her own surgical practice with work on victims of Female Genital Mutilation, chronic vulvar disease like Lichen Sclerosus, reconstruction after vulval cancer, and cosmetic vulval surgery. She is also a member of the British Society for the Study of Vulvar Disease (BSSVD), part of the Cosmetic Committee of the International Society for the Study of Vulval Disease (ISSVD), referent of the Female Genital Mutilation section for the Italian Society of Plastic Surgery (SICPRE), and board of director of the Italian Medical Society of Great Britain (IMSoGB). I met Aurora at a Tony Robbins event in Netherlands and we began a conversation around vaginas. You just never know who you will meet in those events.

My thanks to the women in business in my hometown who signposted me down the right roads; Yvonne Gainford, Sarah McNeill,

Pauline Wright, Sarah Allison, Colette McQueen. To Andrew Armitage of Uber Creative Solutions; he's a creative genie who designed this book cover, etc. and sprinkled his magic over me. Thanks to the local Chamber of Commerce who sent me the prolific author, Paul Teague to guide me past the finishing post of publishing. There has been an Angel waiting for me at every corner of self-doubt and hesitation, I believe he's called Nathan.

To my teachers and mentors, most of whom I haven't met but whose influence has informed and shaped this final trimester of my beautiful and eventful life. My gratitude to Marie Forleo whose B-school is the ultimate in business training for any venture you could dream up. Tony Robbins' programmes leave me breathless and speechless in their depth and breadth, always challenging, exhilarating and fulfilling. Thank you to Magali and Mark Peysha whose RMT school of coaching taught me many of Tony Robbins' skills. Finally, to my son Chris who has been my most exacting teacher and to whom I'm grateful for every conversation.

PS: when you're ready to join a group of positive, happy, and inspirational women who won't settle for less than a fabulous, joyful life, then come along to our Facebookgroup/menopauseunzipped.

Visit www.freddycarrick.com and while there you are welcome to request a simple chart of all Symptoms & Remedies of the menopause and have a browse through the blog posts on up to date information on hormones and all things feminine.

An educational tool for men and another for younger women, plus an online course are all in the pipeline and breaking news will appear on both the above social sites.

ADDITIONAL RESOURCES

Websites:

- The NHS website on HRT: www.nhs.uk
- Prof Klim McPherson: www.obs-gyn.ox.ac.uk
- Prof John Studd: www.studd.co.uk
- The Oxford 'Million Women Study' : www.millionwomenstudy.org
- UK Royal Osteoporosis Society for all information on preventing, recognising and treating poor bone health: www.theros.org.uk
- www.YourPelvicFloor.org.
- British Menopause Society Guidelines: www.thebms.org.uk
- The International Menopause Society (IMS) brings together the world's leading experts to collaborativel study and share knowledge about all aspects of aging in women: www.imsociety.org
- https://www.netdoctor.co.uk/healthy-living/wellbeing/a28594/bioidentical-hormones-menopause-hrt/
- https://www.ncbi.nlm.nih.gov/pubmed/
- MenopauseTaylor hosts a series of educational videos https://www.youtube.com/watch?v=aZ-OaC0KTZE
- UK leading menopause specialist: http://www.drcatherinetupper.co.uk/contact.html
- https://www.news-medical.net/health/Chemical-Classes-Of-Hormones.aspx
- UK mental health charity: www.mind.org.uk
- www.freddycarrick.com
- https://alittlepieceofmind.co.uk a helpful site in support of anyone suffering from anxiety

Clinical trials:

- The Recent Review of the Genitourinary Syndrome of Menopause

Hyun-Kyung Kim et al, published within the Journal of Menopausal Medicine in August 2015, and online August 28th 2015 10.6118/jmm.2015.21.2.65

- Vulvovaginal Atrophy Maire B MacBride, MBBCH, et al. Published within the Mayo Clinic journal in January 2010. Doi: 10.4065/mcp.2009.0413
- Addressing Vulvovaginal Atrophy (VVA)/Genitourinary Syndrome of Menopause (GSM) for Healthy Aging in Women
Rossella E. Nappl et al, published in Frontiers of Endocrinology journal 21st August 2019 and online https://doi.org/10.3389/fendo.2019.00561
Additional research provided by Aurora Almadori ......

TV and YouTube editions:

- Trust Me I'm A Doctor is a BBC TV production https://www.bbc.co.uk/programmes/p01k8vwc
- Dr Louise Newson (GP specialist in menopause) interview https://youtu.be/EwjLP9O1inw
- *Fearless Motivation*, youtube series by Tom Bilyeu, many excellent interviews
- Marie Forleo interview https://youtu.be/ngu3Dcn9F9Y
- Tony Robbins has created a library of YouTube videos and interviews, every single one is golden. Unfortunately,Tony's voice is ragged after 30 odd years of leading huge events, but if you don't mind that, then he's a leader for our times.

Podcasts:

https://www.postcardsfrommidlife.com/
https://tonyrobbins.com/podcasts

Books:

- Alisa Vitti: Woman Code
- Hollie Holden: Notes on Living and Loving
- Gary Chapman: 5 Love Languages
- Marie Forleo: Everything is Figureoutable

- Ray Dalio: Principles
- Gary Renard: The Disappearance of the Universe
- Deepak Chopra: The Mind Body Connection
- Simon Sinek: Start with The Why
- Rick Hanson: Hardwiring Happiness
- Tony Robbins: Unshakeable, Unlimited Power. Everything on his Breakthrough app.
- Brene Brown: I Thought It Was Just Me, Daring Greatly, Dare to Lead
- Glennon Doyle: Untamed
- Elizabeth Gilbert: City of Girls
- Freddy Carrick: Menopause Tracker*, Menopause Journal* Menopause for Men*

(*not yet published but look out for information on www.freddycarrick.com)

INDEX

A

B

C

D

E

F

G

H

I

J

K

L

M

N

O

P

R

S

Printed in Great Britain
by Amazon

44802388R00106